GW00771856

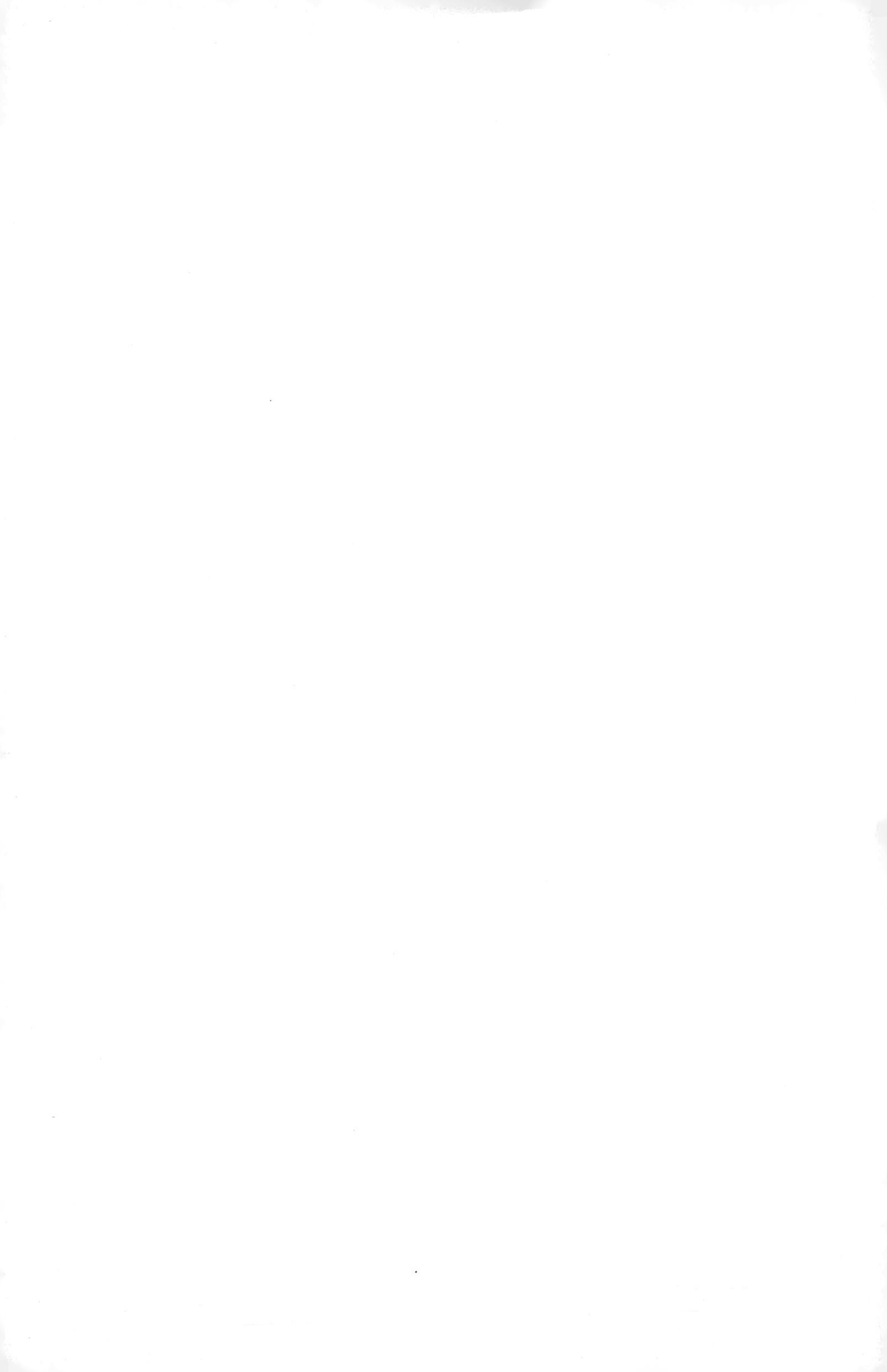

A HISTORY OF THE LEEDS SCHOOL OF MEDICINE

One and a Half Centuries

1831–1981

Leeds School of Medicine.

June 6. 1831.

At a meeting held this day, present Dr. Williamson, Dr. Hunter, Mr. J. Smith, Mr. Wm. Hey, Mr. T. P. Teale, & Mr. Garlick, it was unanimously resolved,

That it is desirable that a School be established in Leeds for the purpose of giving such courses of lectures on subjects connected with Medicine & Surgery as will qualify for examination at the College of Surgeons and Apothecaries' Hall.

That the gentlemen now present do constitute a committee for carrying this project into effect, four of whom shall form a quorum.

That this association be called the "Leeds School of Medicine".

That the expenses of the outfit, and of carrying on the different departments be defrayed out of a fund to which each member of the committee shall equally contribute.

That all receipts be equally divided.

A HISTORY OF THE LEEDS SCHOOL OF MEDICINE

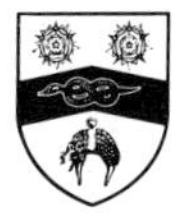

One and a Half Centuries
1831–1981

S. T. ANNING AND W. K. J. WALLS

LEEDS UNIVERSITY PRESS

First published 1982
Reprinted 1993

Leeds School of Medicine

ISBN 0 85316 131 3

Cover illustration
Entrance to the Old Medical School
Architect, W. H. Thorpe, opened 1894
Lithograph by Thomas Hamilton Crawford, 1860–1948
University of Leeds Collections

Printed by LEEDS UNIVERSITY PRESS

Contents

Appendices

List of Illustrations

Foreword

by the

DEAN OF THE FACULTY OF MEDICINE

THE APPROACH of the one hundred and fiftieth session of the Leeds School of Medicine prompted our two colleagues to draw together studies on its earlier history and some account of more recent happenings. Both were well placed to do this because of their sustained interest in the medical history of Leeds, where each has spent most of his professional life.

Stephen Anning came from a Leeds medical family, did his clinical course here and after a period in general practice and the army specialized in dermatology. Successively tutor, clinical lecturer and senior clinical lecturer in that subject he also held the title of Society of Apothecaries' Lecturer in the History of Medicine for many years. Kenneth Walls entered the Medical School in 1934. After qualifying he served in the army and in surgery for a few years before becoming lecturer in anatomy in 1949. Becoming senior lecturer in 1959 he is about to retire this year, after thirty-three years, with an enviable reputation as teacher and friend.

The accounts of successive phases of the School's history are penetrating, well documented and eminently readable. They proceed from its early days in 1831 as a private venture to its present position as a large School in a great civic University. While it will also have an appeal to a wider readership, present and future medical students will find this book fascinating and it will arouse in those who have qualified in medicine here, nostalgic, and no doubt, happy memories of times past.

D. R. Wood

Leeds
1982

Preface

THIS BOOK has been written as a contribution to the celebrations of the 150th anniversary of the founding of the Leeds School. The stimulus for its production must be attributed almost entirely to Dr Stephen Anning who conceived the idea many years ago and kindly invited me to join him.

Over a period of twenty-five years he has studied and written widely on medical history and many of his articles already published have a direct bearing on the history of the Leeds School of Medicine and could properly have been included here. However, in order that the book should take an entirely new look at the history, these have with some regrets on the part of both of us been omitted. However, it will be seen that quotations have been given and reference made to them; they may be consulted elsewhere.

Much new material which has not previously received comment — mainly taken from the minutes and accounts of the School in the independent stage of its existence — has been consulted and appears now for the first time. Hearsay and living memory provide further background. Dr Anning has given help and encouragement to the junior partner throughout and has also been entirely responsible for the index. In any history omissions are inevitable; an attempt to hold the balance has been made and where this has failed the fault is mine. It has been our deliberate policy to keep reference to those at present in post and those still living to a minimum — their turn may come in another fifty years.

We wish to pay tribute to the substantial help, encouragement and forbearance of our wives, Joan and Marguerite, and also wish to thank:
Professor R. L. Holmes, Dr J. A. Sharp, Professor D. R. Wood, Mr William Walls, Mrs Elizabeth Lonsdale, Dr D. Taverner and the late Professor J. M. P. Clark, who have read parts of the manuscript and given useful suggestions;
Dr J. H. Andrew, HM Inspector of Anatomy, for kindly providing copies of early correspondence with the Leeds School of Medicine;
Dr J. MacGregor, Mrs Mary Forster, Mrs R. Stephens and Mrs A. M. Pulleyn for help in making available material from University Archives;
Mrs Mary Forster who also as Librarian of the Thoresby Society, gave help and advice at Claremont;

Mr Martin Julian for access to Planning Bulletins;
Mr Denys Horner for drawing Fig 34 and adding lettering to Figs 3 and 17;
Mr Peter Hargreaves for overall care in the preparation of the illustrations, and his team for their help;
the University Photography Service for provision of negatives for Figs 3, 5, 12, 17, 33, and 35;
Mr E. A. Winstanley of Otley for Fig 36;
Mrs Barbara Whitehead for generous secretarial help and patience in typing the manuscript and to many who, being interested in the history of the School, have contributed in various ways.

A special acknowledgement is due to Mr H. Tolson in particular, and to his colleagues in the University Printing Service, for the wealth of ideas offered, the speedy service and the help given in smoothing the path of publication. Also to the University for providing bridging finance and a limited guarantee against loss. Any profits are to be given to the CL Fund, established in relation to the 150th anniversary.

It is our hope that when the book has been read, Moynihan's remark to students at the time of the Centenary will be understood and echoed by present readers, '*Laetus sorte mea*, the lot is fallen unto me in a fair ground, lo! I have a goodly heritage!'

Leeds
1982

W.K.J.W.

Preface to the Reprint

A REPRINT of the first edition is deemed desirable in view of the interest in the history of the School and in medical education generally. The fact that the changes in the structure and organisation of the School that began in the early 1980s are continuing means that as yet it is too soon to provide a commentary on the development; thus this reprint rather than the addition of supplementary chapters. In a time of rapid change in higher education and the National Health Service a backward look to what are fondly imagined to be more stable times is frequently desired. If it is the hope that this book will provide such a view readers may be disappointed. Financial stringency and competition for scarce resources were constantly facing our forebears, as this admirable work by Kenneth Walls and Stephen Anning makes plain.

The interest in the history of the School is evidenced by the commissioning of a mural depicting its development during its first 150 years. Completed during 1989 by Brian Holmes, the mural is 28ft long and occupies one wall of the Student Common Room in the Worsley Building. The principal benefactor for the mural was the Thackray Medical Research Trust which at the time of publication of this reprint is converting part of Ashley Wing of St James's University Hospital into the Thackray Medical Museum.

It is with sadness that I must record the death of Stephen Anning, co-author of the History, since first publication. The retirement of Kenneth Walls in 1982 has been followed by eleven active years as an Honorary Lecturer to the School.

Leeds
April 1993

William K. Mathie
Secretary to the School of Medicine

CHAPTER ONE

The Setting

THE TRAINING of an apothecary in the late eighteenth and early nineteenth centuries was mainly by apprenticeship, though those who wished to practise generally (surgeon-apothecaries) often added a period 'walking the wards' of a London hospital. The apprenticeship might be for a period of seven or perhaps five years. The apothecaries' licence was obtained by a viva voce examination at Apothecaries Hall, but in 1800 according to Charles Newman, this examination was very sketchy.

For another kind of practitioner, the surgeon, the customary (but not necessary) qualification was membership of the Company of Surgeons, which became the Royal College of Surgeons in 1800. Here the emphasis lay more heavily on anatomy since in pre-anaesthetic days speed of operating was essential and the relations of organs needed to be known. Hospital experience of six months (increased in 1813 to one year) was also required, but medicine was not examined.[1]

The training can be exemplified by that of William Hey (the first) who in 1767 helped to found the Leeds General Infirmary. In 1750 at the age of fourteen he was bound apprentice for seven years to William Dawson, surgeon-apothecary of Leeds. The indenture of 24 June witnessed to this and continued 'During all of which Term, the said Apprentice his said Master well and faithfully shall serve, his Secrets shall keep, his lawful Commands shall do, Fornication or Adultery shall not commit, Hurt or Damage to his said Master shall not do, or Consent to be done, but to his Power shall Lett it, and forthwith his said Master thereof warn: Taverns or Ale-Houses he shall not Haunt or Frequent, unless it be about his Master's Business there to be done: At Dice, Cards, Tables, Bowls or any other unlawful Games he shall not Play: The Goods of his Master he shall not waste nor them Lend, or give to any Person without his Master's Licence: Matrimony with any woman within the Term shall not contract, nor from his Master's Service at any time absent himself; but as a True and Faithful Apprentice shall Order and behave himself towards his said Master, and all as well in Words as in Deeds, during the said Term: and a True and just Account of all his said Master's Goods Chattles and Money committed to his Charge, or which shall come into his Hands, Faithfully he shall give at all Times when thereunto required by his said Master, his Executors, Administrators or Assigns. AND the said William Dawson for and in consideration of the Sum of Thirty Pounds of Good and lawful money of Great Britain' . . . promised to . . . 'Teach, Learn and Inform his said Apprentice . . . in the Arts Trades or Mysteries of an Apothecary and Surgeon . . . AND also shall find, provide to and for his the said Apprentice, sufficient and enough of Meat Drink and Lodging, and also Wash for his said Apprentice two shirts weekly during the said Term.'[2] Apprenticeship often involved menial tasks, such as sweeping out the surgery and its value depended much on the excellence and conscientiousness of the Master. At the end of the apprenticeship Hey went to London for two years: first, six months' dissection, then on to St George's Hospital to study under William Bromfield, whose pupil and later dresser he became. He also attended lectures on medicine and midwifery.

There was another class of practitioner, namely the physicians. Theirs was an academic training. They went to a University, commonly Edinburgh, Leyden, Oxford or Cambridge, and were well educated in the classics to which a variable amount of vocational material was added for the MD degree. They were trained to be thinkers and counsellors rather than skilled craftsmen — often it is said they did not examine their patients.

The first six physicians at the Leeds Infirmary, spanning the years 1767 to 1833 had become Doctors of Medicine of either Edinburgh or Leyden, where at that time were the foremost medical faculties in Europe.

The only hospital medical schools in London in 1800 were at St Bartholomew's, St Thomas's, Guy's and the London. Elsewhere students were able to attend hospital practice, but times were restricted, eg 10 am to 2 pm and so they often attended more than one hospital in trying to make up their programme. The situation was unsatisfactory. Private schools of Anatomy grew up and flourished.

In the early nineteenth century there was a growing awareness that professional training could be improved by making it more systematic and self regulation in the professions was already under way. The advancement of science meant more knowledge in botany, chemistry and in due course in physiology to be added to the curriculum.

The passing of the Apothecaries' Act of 1815, which gave the Society of Apothecaries powers of examination and of the issue of licences, added a further stimulus to the development of provincial medical schools.

In Leeds at the Infirmary anatomical demonstrations had been given on the bodies of criminals executed at York: the first in 1773 and then by William Hey in 1800, 1803, 1805, and 1809.[3] The last was on Mary Bateman, the 'Yorkshire Witch', who had been systematically robbing Rebecca Perigo and her husband. When they were beginning to complain she had provided them with a poisoned pudding and Rebecca Perigo had died.[4] Mary Bateman's skeleton is still to be found in the Museum in the Department of Anatomy and is interesting because of the presence of a cervical rib. These demonstrations, however useful, were too few and far between to provide for the needs of medical students.

The next development of note came in the 1820s. Charles Turner Thackrah an apothecary-surgeon enjoyed teaching and by 1821 had already acquired six apprentices. The teaching which he offered grew into the Leeds School of Anatomy which he established in his own house in South Parade in late 1826 or early 1827.[5]

The population of Leeds and the surrounding villages in 1831 was approaching 100,000.[6] The Leeds, York and Clothing District Directory for 1830 lists seven physicians and forty-seven surgeons resident in the Leeds district. The medical institutions already established in the town were five in number:

1. The Infirmary in Infirmary Street with gardens running down to Wellington Street.
2. The Dispensary in North Street.
3. The House of Recovery, fever hospital in Vicar Lane.
4. The Eye and Ear Infirmary at 115 Kirkgate.
5. The Lying-in Hospital in St Peter's Square.

The Infirmary, the Dispensary and the House of Recovery were each staffed by three physicians and three surgeons some of whom served more than one institution.[7]

The advantages of a provincial medical school over its London counterparts may be summarised from an early prospectus: 'greater facilities of seeing hospital practice, in consequence of the smaller number of Pupils, — a more intimate association with the several Teachers, — and exemption from those sources of distraction and dissipation, peculiar to a great capital. The benefits resulting from the vigilant superintendence of the Master, over the moral habits of his Pupil, are conjoined with a plan of academic study, and the student is enabled to qualify himself for the active exercise of his profession, under the immediate observation of his relations and friends.'[8]

London schools were overcrowded; distance from the schools of London, Edinburgh, Glasgow, Aberdeen and Dublin and slowness of travel made provincial schools convenient. The time was ripe for the development of another provincial school.

REFERENCES

1. Charles Newman, *The evolution of Medical Education in the Nineteenth Century*, London, 1957.
2. J. B. Hellier, *On the history of Medical Education in Leeds — an address for Students Medical Society in the Library, Leeds School of Medicine*, 1921, Typescript, Leeds Reference Library.
3. S. T. Anning, *The History of Medicine in Leeds*, Leeds, 1980.
4. *The New Newgate Calendar*, Ed Lord Birkett, London, 1960, pp 35–47.
5. H. Y. Whytehead, *Biographical Memoir of C. T. Thackrah* 1834, quoted in A. Meiklejohn, *Thackrah Anthology*, 1957, unpublished, in Medical Library, University of Leeds.
6. Wm. White, *History and General Directory of Leeds*, Sheffield, 1837, p 478.
7. *Directory of the Borough of Leeds, the City of York and the Clothing District of Yorkshire*, Leeds, 1830.
8. Leeds School of Medicine, Prospectus 1834.

CHAPTER TWO

The Foundation

AT LEAST ten provincial medical schools arose in the decade 1824–34.[1]

In 1831 there were already medical schools in Manchester, Birmingham, Sheffield, Newcastle upon Tyne, and Norwich. Practitioners, apprentices and public opinion generally favoured such a development in Leeds.[2] Thackrah felt it strongly for his School of Anatomy, already almost five years old, had not become recognised by the College of Surgeons.[3] Thackrah was not however present at the meeting which instituted the school of medicine but became involved a few days later.

The minutes of the initial meeting, the first page of which is shown in the frontispiece, may be quoted in full:

> 'Leeds School of Medicine
> June 6, 1831
>
> At a meeting held this day, present Dr Williamson, Dr Hunter, Mr S. Smith, Mr Wm. Hey, Mr T. P. Teale and Mr Garlick, it was unanimously resolved,
>
> That it is desirable that a School be established in Leeds for the purpose of giving such courses of lectures on subjects connected with Medicine & Surgery as will qualify for examination at the College of Surgeons and Apothecaries' Hall.
>
> That the gentlemen now present do constitute a committee for carrying this project into effect, four of whom shall form a quorum.
>
> That this association be called the "Leeds School of Medicine".
>
> That the expenses of the outfit and of carrying on the different departments be defrayed out of a fund to which each member of the committee shall equally contribute.
>
> That all receipts be equally divided.
>
> That each member of the committee having expressed his willingness to give lectures on some particular branch of medical science be considered as appointed to the respective departments as follows:

Principles & Practice of Physic	Dr Williamson
Materia Medica and Therapeutics	Dr Hunter
Operative Surgery	Mr S. Smith

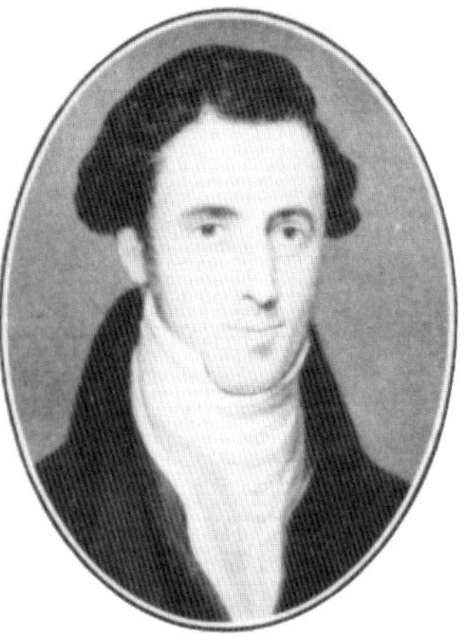

JAMES WILLIAMSON
6 June 1831

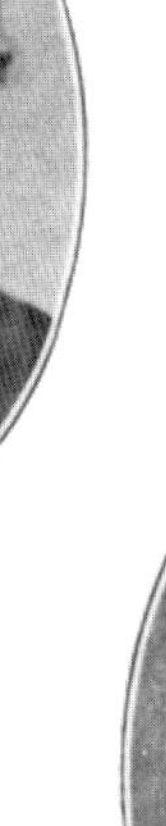

THOMAS PRIDGIN TEALE
6 June 1831
(Secretary)

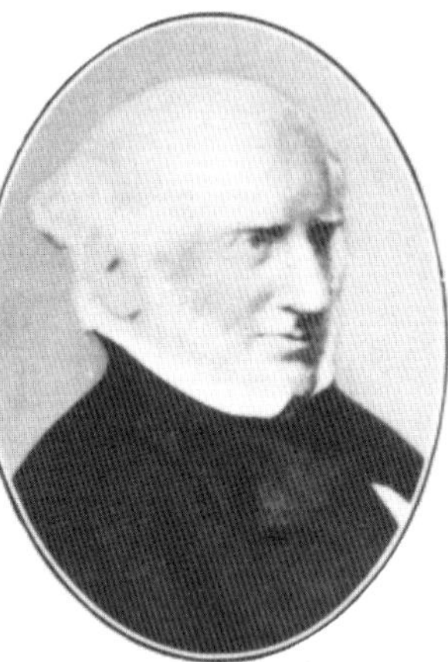

JOSEPH PRINCE GARLICK
6 June 1831
(Treasurer)

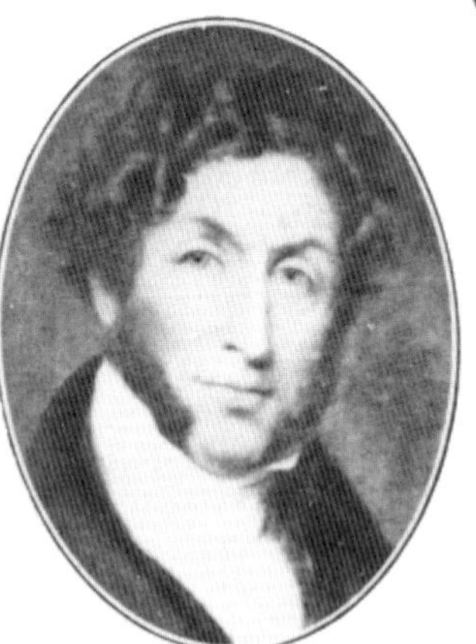

ADAM HUNTER
6 June 1831

FIG. 1 *Founders*

Midwifery & Diseases of Women & Children	Mr S. Smith
Principles & Practice of Surgery	Mr Wm. Hey
Anatomy & Physiology	Mr T. P. Teale and Mr Garlick

That Wm. Hey Esqre be invited to allow his name to appear as a lecturer and to take a part of any of the anatomical or surgical lectures which he may choose.

That Dr Disney Thorp be invited to cooperate with the committee and that one of the departments of Chemistry, Botany or Forensic Medicine be offered to him.

That no future appointment shall be made except by an unanimous vote of the committee.

That Mr T. P. Teale be appointed Secretary.'[4]

Of those who attended this meeting two were physicians to both the Infirmary and the Dispensary, two were surgeons to the Infirmary and two were surgeons to the Dispensary.

A biographer in 1831 might have described them thus:

Dr James Williamson was born in Chester in 1797 and so is 34 or thereabouts; he lives at 4 Park Square; he was elected physician to the Infirmary in February 1824 and also physician to the Dispensary from the time of its foundation in June of the same year; he is a gentleman of some personal means, professional, dignified, courteous and helpful and will have a moderating effect on others.

Dr Adam Hunter is 37 and has been living at 10 Park Row but is moving to 48 Park Square. He wrote in 1819 an essay on *Two Mineral Springs of Harrogate and the Springs of Thorp Arch and Ilkley* and more recently *A Treatise on the Waters of Harrogate*; he was joint secretary with Thackrah of the Leeds Philosophical and Literary Society from 1819 to 1822. He has been physician to both Infirmary and Dispensary for seven years, haveing been appointed to both in June 1824; he will be remembered for the tenacity with which he holds his opinions.

Samuel Smith, MRCS Eng. (1812), the oldest of the group is aged 41; born in Leeds he was apprenticed to his brother-in-law, Thomas Fawell, an apothecary-surgeon who practised in Commercial Street; he continued his studies in London under Sir Charles Bell and in Edinburgh. He is athletic and has a robust constitution. He was elected surgeon to the Infirmary in 1819 and now lives at 8 Park Row; a man well endowed with common sense; alive to and active against social evils, eg long hours of work by children in mills and pits.

William Hey (the third), MRCS Eng. (1818), is 35; practises at 36 Albion Street on the corner with Albion Place in a house* with two acres of garden, built by his grandfather William Hey (the first): he was elected surgeon to the Infirmary last December, 1830, on the retirement of his father William Hey (the second).

Thomas Pridgin Teale, MRCS Eng. (1823), is 30, the eldest son of a Leeds practitioner. Educated at Heath Grammar School, Halifax and Leeds Grammar School, he spent short periods at Leeds Infirmary and in Edinburgh and then three winters at the United Hospitals in London, St Thomas's and Guy's, before being elected surgeon to the Dispensary in 1824. He lives at 22 Albion Street and his interests extend to zoology, geology and salmon fishing. Like the first William Hey he lost an eye in childhood. It is said that at the age of 22 he became the first provincial surgeon to tie the subclavian artery for axillary aneurysm.

Joseph Prince Garlick, MRCS Eng. LSA (1817), is 38, was apothecary to the Infirmary 1815–22, where also his sister was matron for nine years from 1817. He has been surgeon to the Dispensary since 1824 and though not on the medical staff of the Infirmary he has been a member of the Weekly Board since 1828; he helped to found the West Riding Medical Charitable Society in 1829 and is its secretary. His home is at 21 Park Row.[5]

So the School was established quietly, not by a meeting of the nobility and gentry, nor by public subscription, but by six relatively young and active men, who possessed a certain spirit of independence and self reliance. Of the invitations which they issued at the first meeting one was to a senior colleague, Mr William Hey's father, and was not taken up. He had lately retired from the Infirmary and was to be Mayor of Leeds for the ensuing year. The other was to a man younger than themselves Disney Launder Thorp, MD, born in 1805, whose father was the senior of the Infirmary's three physicians.

At the second meeting, held at Dr Williamson's house four days after the first, Dr Disney Thorp had joined the committee and had chosen the Department of Forensic Medicine, to which he was there and then appointed. An advertisement was then drafted for insertion in the Leeds newspapers, which indicated that lectures would start in November (later advanced to 25 October) and listed the various subjects and lecturers, declared that arrangements were in the making for courses on

* The house is still standing and is presently the Law Society Office, near the Leeds Club in Albion Place.

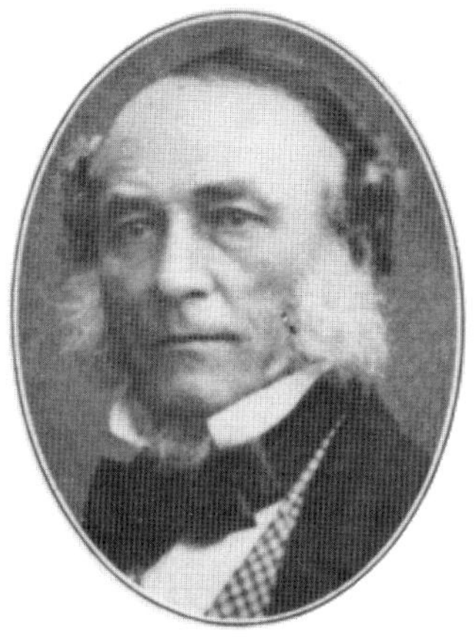

WILLIAM HEY
6 June 1831

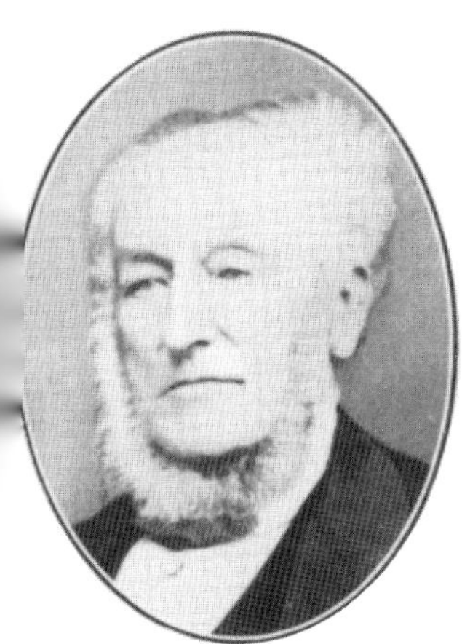

SAMUEL SMITH
6 June 1831

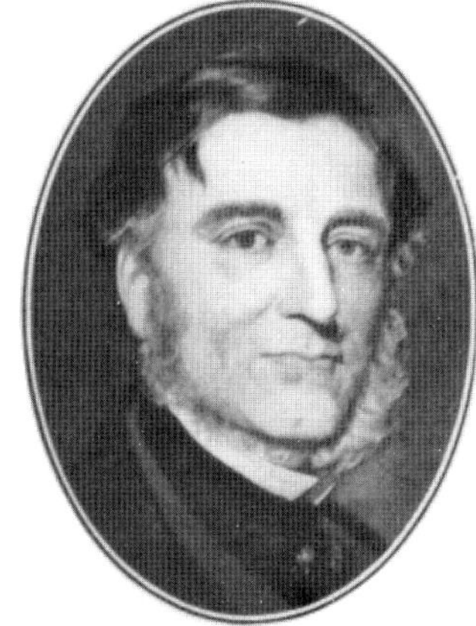

DISNEY LAUNDER THORP
10 June 1831

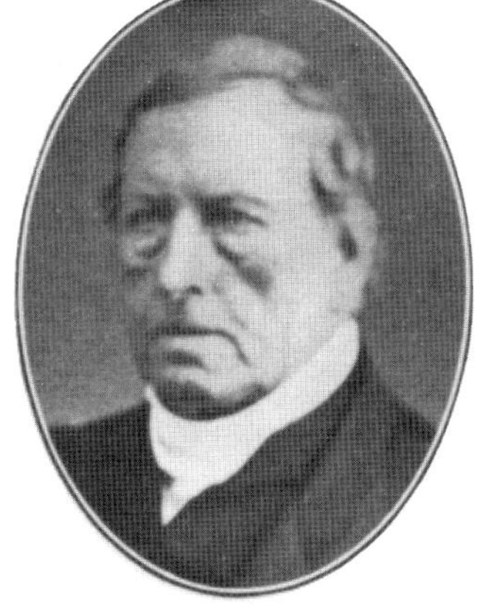

WILLIAM PRICE
26 July 1831

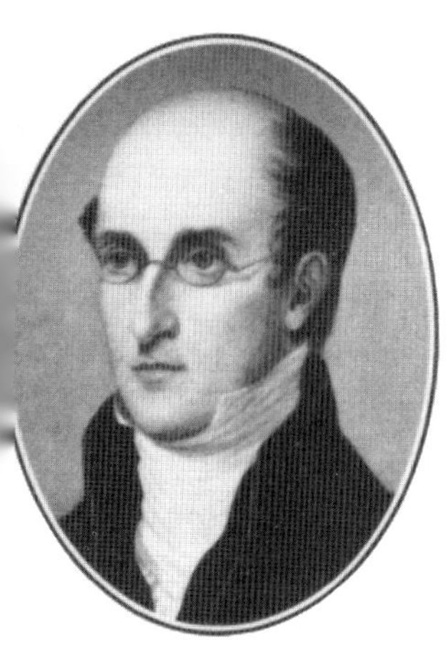

CHARLES TURNER THACKRAH
14 June 1831

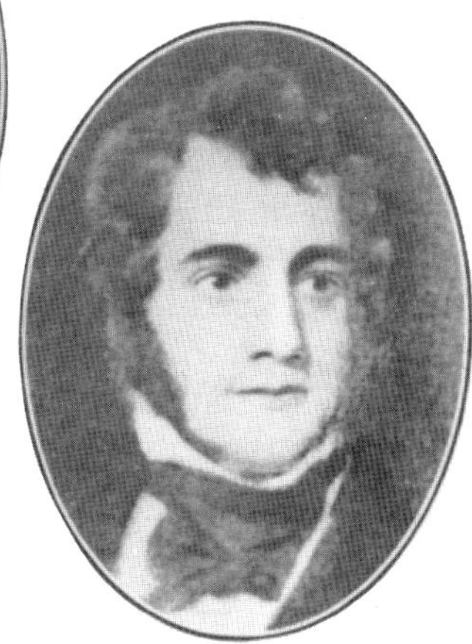

JOHN HEY
19 August 1831

FIG. 2 *Founders*

chemistry and botany and added that 'the entire series will be adapted to the regulations of the College of Surgeons and Society of Apothecaries'.[6]

The following day, 11 June, the third meeting was held at Mr Garlick's and resolved 'that Mr Thackrah be invited to cooperate with the committee and that a deputation wait upon him to request his attendance at this meeting'. Such a resolution was possible since Mr Thackrah lived a mere 200 yards away at 9 South Parade. The deputation must have found him at home for the minutes of the meeting continue: 'That as Mr Thackrah accepts the invitation of the committee the following addition be made to the advertisement "Mr Thackrah will take a part in the anatomical and surgical courses."'[7]

Charles Turner Thackrah, LSA, MRCS Eng (1816) was in private practice. Born in Leeds in 1795 he was apprenticed to a Leeds practitioner, had become a student of the Infirmary in 1814 and had spent the winter of 1815–16 at Guy's Hospital under Sir Astley Cooper. He was able and active, worked long hours despite ill health and had several well-received publications to his credit. These were mainly on the blood, on philosophy and on social conditions. He had become interested in teaching, had given a series of popular lectures on physiology and as previously noted had set up a private school of anatomy in his own home. He had publicly quarrelled with the Infirmary doctors in 1827,[8] in a letter to the *Leeds Mercury* calling them 'The Arrogants' and 'Backbiters' and complaining of their treatment of his pupils and himself. Sam Smith replied naming him 'Mr Puff' and detailing the reasons why the respectable part of the profession did not wish to associate with him.[9] But after his second marriage in 1829 relationships had improved and now he and the others would find association in the School of Medicine of mutual benefit.

Much needed to be done and many arrangments made if the School was to open in the autumn and something of the urgency of the situation is captured by following the minutes of the nineteen meetings of the committee held in the four and a half months that intervened. Most of these meetings were held in the houses of the members in rotation and at first the Chairmanship also rotated but after the ninth meeting on 26 July, it seemed natural for Dr Williamson to take the Chair. It was at this meeting also that the committee is first referred to as the Council. On 14 June Mr Thackrah was deputed to 'make application to the Society of Apothecaries for recognition of the different lecturers' and it was decided to invite Mr William Price, an ex-naval surgeon, to give lectures on Military Surgery and Mr Cass, the only other surgeon to the Dispensary at that time to take the course of Botany.[10] Mr Cass declined.

Later in the month an approach was made to Mr William West, a chemist with a business in Briggate, to give lectures on Chemistry,[11] and on 2 July Mr West's proposal was accepted, that he give '45 lectures of an hour each, for half a guinea each lecture and one guinea for each pupil — Mr West to provide the apparatus and materials'.[12] Mr West, 'a member of the Society of Friends, of rather eccentric habits, distinguished for active benevolence', continued to lecture for sixteen years, was elected FRS but was never a member of the Council.

Premises were needed for the School and it seemed that the Dispensary, which had been founded in 1824 at the House of Recovery in Vicar Lane near to the junction with Kirkgate and had moved in 1828 to its own building in North Street,[13] had spare capacity. The Annual Meeting of the Dispensary was due on 7 July and Dr Williamson and Mr Garlick were to make application 'for the use of certain rooms upon such terms as the annual meeting shall deem suitable'. It seemed that two demonstrators would be desirable, 'to give 4 or 5 demonstrations weekly from 10 to 11 am and supervise dissections from 11 to 12 am'[14] and on 26 July Mr Henry Bell was appointed 'to assist more particularly in the anatomical department and also as far as practicable in the other arrangements of the School'. He would be paid a 'salary of eighty pounds for one year, enter his duties on the 1st of October next. He will be required to lodge in the house (a room to be provided by the Council which is to be furnished by himself), and will be expected to devote his whole time to the school subject to the arrangements of the council.'[15] It was the first whole time appointment. At the same meeting Mr William Price was elected Senior Demonstrator and a member of the Council.

Portraits, some taken in later life, of the founders of the School, are shown in Figs 1 and 2.

The meeting on 30 July was held at the Dispensary. The annual meeting of the Dispensary had called a special general meeting, by advertisement, for 28 July and this had resolved 'That the whole of the north wing of the Dispensary with the exception of the waiting room and surgery be let to the Leeds School of Medicine at the annual rent of ten pounds, with permission to make such arrangements as may render it suitable for the use of that school and to build over the coach house at any future period if necessary.' Dr Williamson, Mr Garlick and Mr Thackrah were to arrange the necessary alterations to the building and Mr Garlick was appointed Treasurer of the School.[16] A plumber, a joiner and a bricklayer were employed and the alterations cost a total of £60.

The Dispensary building fronted on to North Street (now Vicar Lane) on a site presently occupied by the Jumbo Restaurant and close to the corner with Templar Street. It lay opposite to and between the entry of Merrion Street and the Grammar School of that day and close to what is now the West Yorkshire bus station. The rooms in the north wing would abut on the back of the Templar Inn and so would receive their light from the Dispensary courtyard, itself entered from a cul-de-sac off North Street known as North Court. From the Ordnance Survey of 1850 reproduced opposite, there would appear to be six or seven rooms on the north side though perhaps only three or four (per floor) in the north wing abutting on the courtyard.[17] One room must have been used for lectures and we know from later minutes that amongst other rooms were a dissecting room, a laboratory and a museum, which latter was also considered as the private room of the lecturers and 'in their absence it be used by Mr Bell as his sitting room'.[18]

During August it was arranged that Mr John Hey would undertake the department of Botany, in conjunction with Mr Denny, and would become a member of Council.[19] John Hey was the second son of William Hey (the second) and was a surgeon with wide interests in natural science but especially in botany and geology. The Society of Apothecaries replied favourably to the request for recognition and the Council went on to fix the fees for attendance upon the different lectures.

	First course	Second course	Perpetual
Anat^y	4–4–0	3–3–0	8–8–0
Demonst	2–2–0	1–1–0	—
Surgery Oper^ve Surgery }	3–3–0	—	5–5–0
Materia Medica	2–2–0	—	4–4–0
Chemistry	2–2–0	—	—
Physic	3–3–0	—	5–5–0
Midwifery	3–3–0	2–2–0	6–6–0
Botany	1–1–0	—	—
Forensic Medicine	1–1–0	—	—

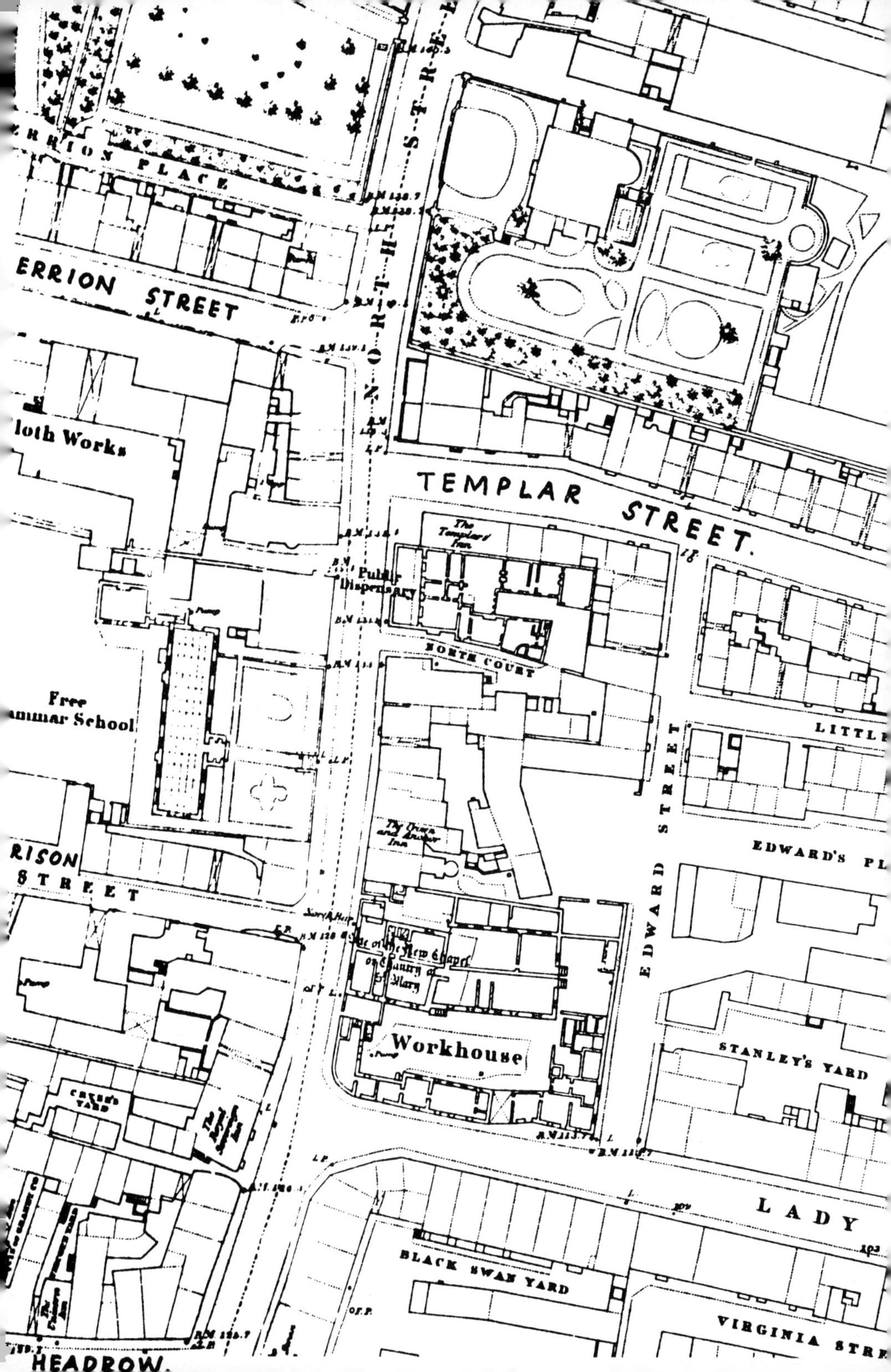

RRION PLACE
NORTH STREET
ERRION STREET
loth Works
TEMPLAR STREET
The Templars Inn
Public Dispensary
NORTH COURT
Free
ammar School
LITTLE
RISON
STREET
The Crown and Anchor Inn
EDWARD STREET
EDWARD'S PL
Site of the New Chapel or Chantry of St. Mary
Workhouse
STANLEY'S YARD
LADY
BLACK SWAN YARD
VIRGINIA STRE
HEADROW.

A prospectus was printed and circulated to the medical practitioners of the West Riding with the exception of the Sheffield District. A second edition of 500 copies was required and these were sent 'to the clergy & to gentlemen in the profession of the law & left at the booksellers, newsrooms, libraries etc. in Leeds'.[20]

The Leeds Mercury of Saturday, 27 August 1831, reported:

> 'We are gratified to find that the Leeds School of Medicine, the project of which we some time since noticed, is to commence its operations on the 25th of October — the names of the physicians and surgeons who have undertaken the several courses of lectures are a guarantee of the respectability of the school; and we anticipate that its establishment will be of much advantage to young men passing through their apprenticeship in this town, as well as a means of raising still higher the profession amongst us. We make the following extract from the prospectus of the School of Medicine:
>
> "It may naturally excite surprise, that while every great town on the Continent of Europe, and in the United States of America, has long since possessed a medical school — in England, with the exception of the Metropolis the formation of such institutions should be of recent origin. The period has at length arrived when both the altered circumstances of society and growing intelligence and respectability of the medical profession (requiring corresponding efforts to sustain them) seem to call for the establishment of provincial schools whenever the population and consequently the number of practitioners are large . . . It is time then that Leeds, the fifth town of England, the centre of a most important and populous district, possessing also in its large and various public medical Establishments, peculiar facilities for the study and illustration of disease — should be able to enumerate amongst its beneficial institutions, one subservient to the cultivation of the medical sciences.
>
> "To achieve an object so desirable, the several Physicians and Surgeons whose names are annexed, have associated themselves into a school, where the various subjects included in the ordinary scheme of medical education may be taught. In the arrangements necessary to organise the institution public utility has been consulted rather than individual interests and predilections and the hours of lectures will be so appointed as to interfere as little as possible with the domestic and professional regulations of masters. Accommodation for the proposed school has been secured in apartments belonging to the Dispensary and it is confidently hoped that the Council will soon be able to announce that their certificates will be received by the Royal College of Surgeons and the Worshipful Company of Apothecaries.

> "With these advantages it is presumed, the Leeds School of Medicine, may prove useful to those within its immediate sphere, not only for facilitating their earliest studies, but also by superseding, or materially abridging the term of residence in London, often inconvenient by its length and expensiveness"[21]

In early October it was decided that the 'anatomical season comprize two courses of 70 lectures each', and agreed that Military and Naval Medical Officers should have gratuitous admission. Resident medical practitioners were to be admitted to the courses on the same terms as other pupils but to individual lectures at the courtesy of the lecturers. A glass case (£15) and other requisites were purchased and there was a call for an instalment of £5 from each member of Council, to be paid to the Treasurer.[22] Arrangements were made for the cleaning of the rooms: 'that the boy, now engaged at the Dispensary, be employed in the dissecting room at the rate of one guinea per quarter during the session'[23] and it was agreed to pay Mr and Mrs Hopwood £6 per annum for the assistance of their servant in cleaning the remainder of the premises and for Mr Hopwood's occasional assistance.[24]

The plan of the Lectures (Fig 4) was published in the *Lancet*, *Medical Gazette*, *Leeds Mercury* and the *Leeds Intelligencer*. Above this advertisement in the *Leeds Mercury* of 15 October, is found another notice:

'LEEDS SCHOOL OF ANATOMY — MR THACKRAH begs to state that having taken a Part in the Leeds School of Medicine, the School of Anatomy conducted by him for the last Five Winters will be suspended, and that the Gentlemen who had Perpetual Admission to his Lectures will have the same to the Anatomical Lectures of the Leeds School of Medicine

South Parade Oct — 13, 1831.'[25]

The School of Medicine opened as planned on 25 October and the following account is taken in abridged form from the *Leeds Mercury* of Saturday, 29 October 1831:

'We had the gratification to attend the opening of the Leeds School of Medicine on Tuesday last . . .

'The Introductory Lecture was to have been delivered by DR WILLIAMSON, but owing to the indisposition of that gentleman, his lecture was postponed and the honourable task of opening the Leeds School of Medicine was assigned to MR THOS. PRIDGIN TEALE. That gentleman executed the duty in a manner most able and satisfactory. He developed

LEEDS SCHOOL OF MEDICINE, DISPENSARY, North-Street.—The FIRST SESSION WILL COMMENCE ON TUESDAY, 25th October, 1831, in which the following COURSES OF LECTURES will be delivered.

ANATOMY, PHYSIOLOGY, and PATHOLOGY, by Mr. T. P. TEALE, and Mr. GARLICK.

The LECTURES on the THORACIC VISCERA, by Mr. THACKRAH.

Tuesday, Wednesday, Thursday, Friday, and Saturday, at Twelve o'Clock.

The Introductory Lecture will be given on Tuesday, Oct. 25, at Twelve o'Clock.

DEMONSTRATIONS and DISSECTIONS, by Mr. PRICE, and Mr. HENRY BELL.

Regularly at Ten a.m.

PRINCIPLES and PRACTICE of SURGERY, by Mr. WILLIAM HEY.

The LECTURES on HERNIA, and on the DISEASES of the PELVIC VISCERA, by Mr. THACKRAH.

OPERATIVE SURGERY, by Mr. SMITH and Mr. WILLIAM HEY.

Tuesday, Thursday, and Saturday, at Seven p.m.

The Introductory Lecture, Tuesday, Oct. 25, Seven p.m.

MATERIA MEDICA, and THERAPEUTICS, by Dr. HUNTER.

Monday and Wednesday, at Seven p.m.

The Introductory Lecture, Wednesday, Oct. 26, Seven p.m.

CHEMISTRY, by Mr. WEST.

Tuesday and Thursday, at Eight p.m.

The Introductory Lecture, Thursday, Oct. 27, Eight p.m.

PRINCIPLES and PRACTICE of PHYSIC, by Dr. WILLIAMSON.

Monday and Wednesday, at Eight p.m.

The Introductory Lecture, Wednesday, Oct. 26, Eight p.m.

BOTANY, by Mr. JOHN HEY, and Mr. DENNY.

In the Summer Months.

FORENSIC MEDICINE, by Dr. DISNEY THORP.

Tuesday, Seven p.m.

MIDWIFERY, and DISEASES of WOMEN and CHILDREN, by Mr. SMITH.

Monday and Thursday, at Seven a.m.

The Introductory Lecture, Thursday, Oct. 27, Seven a.m.

Clinical Lectures will be given gratuitously, to the Pupils of the Infirmary and Dispensary; the Terms of Attendance on the Medical and Surgical Practice of these Institutions may be ascertained by applying to the Resident Medical Officers of each. The Certificates for such Attendance qualify for Examination at the College of Surgeons and Apothecaries' Hall.

***Those intending to enter to the respective Classes, are requested to apply for Tickets, to Mr. Garlick, 21, Park Row, of whom may be procured the Prospectus of the School, announcing the Fees for Attendance upon Lectures.
Leeds, Oct. 11, 1831.

FIG. 4 *Courses of Lectures in the First Session, 1831*

the objects and plan of the institution in a luminous statement and illustrated the advantages of a provincial school of medicine — showing that they were in some respects superior to those of the metropolitan schools. He then addressed a few words of counsel — equally just and impressive — to the young students; after which he commenced his own course of lectures on Anatomy, Physiology and Pathology (which he delivers in conjunction with Mr Thackrah and Mr Garlick) by remarks on Inorganic and Organic Matter, on Animate Bodies Vitality and Nutrition; on Vegetables and Animals. The Lecture was characterised by great purity of taste and elegance of language, as well as by Justice of thought, elevated views and correct knowledge.

'The lecture-room, which is at the Dispensary, was quite filled on the occasion; most of the principal professional gentlemen of the town were present as well as the medical students and a few non professional visitors. The lecture was received with merited applause.'

The *Mercury* did not exaggerate. Mr Teale developed his argument well and many of his general statements would be equally true and applicable if made today, one hundred and fifty years later. He said 'It must be admitted that science . . . has of late made great advances and in some of the departments has even far exceeded the most sanguine anticipations of our immediate predecessors.' Men would wish to see their own departments at least keep pace with others and 'the Committee consider that they cannot in any way more effectively promote the medical sciences than by improving the means of medical education.

'That many glaring defects exist in the present system is acknowledged by all who are in the least conversant with it and although they may not at present admit of being entirely removed yet much may now be done towards amelioration.' He notes that the time usually allotted to medical education in England and Wales is seven years; five in apprenticeship and the last two in attending lectures and hospitals in London. He points out that the two great disadvantages of this scheme are the hitherto unavoidable absence of a regular or systematic course of study during apprenticeship and the consequent overcrowding of lectures in all subjects into the short space of two years. 'By the establishment of provincial schools these defects will be greatly rectified. Facilities will thus be afforded for more equally distributing the various branches of study throughout the entire period of education . . . Habits of order and regularity will be acquired; the mind will be early trained in observation:

facts of importance, which daily present themselves, will be fully appreciated.

'No one will deny the advantage of devoting a period of *seven* years to the deliberate study of Anatomy, Physiology, and Pathology, Surgery, Materia Medica, Physic, Botany, Forensic Medicine, Midwifery, — instead of condensing into the short space of two years the required number of courses:— under which system the student has to hurry from one lecture to another, with but little time for reflection and study, or for the practical application of what he has heard.'

Mr Teale went on to show that the study of Anatomy did not require to be done in the metropolis, pointing out the number of towns in Germany and Italy which possessed schools of anatomy and that many of the best examinees at the Society of Apothecaries were from the provinces; nor did the study of Chemistry, instancing the name of Dalton; nor did clinical work — provincial practitioners 'need not cede priority to their highly gifted brethren of the metropolis . . . Hospitals of many of the large towns of England afford greater advantages than those of London — for this simple reason; that the number of pupils is much more limited. Each case is accessible to every pupil, whereas of the crowds that run through the wards of a metropolitan institution how few are there who can obtain a transient glance at the patient.' Leeds with its Infirmary, House of Recovery, Dispensary and Lying-in Hospital presents excellent opportunities for clinical instruction. 'The committee . . . have the satisfaction to announce that since the publication of their prospectus they have been favoured with letters from the Royal College of Surgeons and the Worshipful Society of Apothecaries expressive of their approbation and conveying the promise, that after the different courses have been completed, the certificates of attendance upon such courses will receive their recognition.'

Mr Teale then gave his advice to the students:

'There are certain errors which I particularly wish to guard you against at the commencement of your career.

'It is too frequently considered by the medical student that the *great end* of his studies is to qualify himself for passing an examination and obtaining a diploma.

'Let me beg of you to aim at nobler objects. Let your unwearied endeavours be to store the mind, not merely for passing an examination, but for future usefulness.

'Permit me also to guard you against the too prevalent idea on receiving a diploma or what is termed "completing your education" that you have exhausted the stores of science, — that nothing more is to be learnt, — that you are infallible. Every subsequent part of your life will convince you of your delusion. Indeed so far from the act of receiving a diploma being considered the *completion* of your medical education you must regard it as being the *very threshold* —The whole life of a medical practitioner is one continued course of pupilage.

'It was remarked by one of the brightest ornaments of our profession . . . that each succeeding year convinced him more and more how little knowledge he possessed.

'These remarks are offered with a two-fold view:—

'1st. To check the satisfaction which so sadly may beset the student, on emerging from the schools, and which cannot fail to check his advance of knowledge and consequently to diminish his usefulness.

'2ndly. To hold out an inducement for steady perseverence in careful observation and reflection, since the whole extent of science is not compassed during the academic routine, but regions unexplored still remain to invite the steps of the patient investigator and will not fail to repay him abundantly with a rich and luxurious harvest.

'Let me now seriously entreat you to consider well the aweful responsibilities you are taking upon yourselves: that being deeply impressed with the important part you have to perform, you may eagerly grasp every opportunity for storing the mind with valuable information.

'The influence of your education is not limited to yourselves or to your own domestic circles:— It extends throughout society, — You may be a blessing or a curse to thousands. Under divine Providence, you will often be the arbiters of life and death. Oft you will hold the balance, and through your instrumentality, the beam may turn to life and joy, — or to death and woe.

'Let there then be engraven on your mind, in characters too deep to be effaced "*Orphan — Widow*". Think of the ties your ignorance will dissever:— Think of the blessings your honest industry may diffuse.'[26]

REFERENCES

1. S. T. Anning, *The History of Medicine in Leeds*, Leeds, 1980, p 135.
2. Prospectus Leeds School of Medicine, quoted by *Leeds Mercury*, 27 August 1831.

3. S. T. Anning, op cit, p 147.
4. Leeds School of Medicine Council Book 1, 6 June 1831.
5. Biographical notes taken from
   R. V. Taylor, *Biographia Leodiensis*, London, 1865
   S. T. Anning, *The General Infirmary at Leeds*, vol II, Edinburgh and London, 1966, Appendix III
   W. N. Price, *Introductory Address 1881*, Leeds School of Medicine Prospectuses 1864-84, in Medical Library, University of Leeds
   J. B. Hellier, *On the history of Medical Education in Leeds — an address for Students Medical Society in the Library, Leeds School of Medicine*, 1921, Typescript, Leeds Reference Library.
   Lord Moynihan, 'Days Gone By', *University of Leeds Medical Society Magazine*, Vol IV, 1934, pp 36–7.
   General and Commercial Directory of the Borough of Leeds, 1826.
   Leeds York and Clothing Directory, 1830.
6. Leeds School of Medicine Council Book 1, 10 June 1831.
7. Ibid, 11 June 1831.
8. A. Meiklejohn, *Thackrah Anthology* 1957.
9. *Leeds Mercury* 19 May 1827, 26 May 1827, 1 June 1827.
10. Leeds School of Medicine Council Book 1, 14 June 1831.
11. Ibid, 25 June 1831.
12. Ibid, 2 July 1831.
13. S. T. Anning, *The History of Medicine in Leeds*, Leeds, 1980, p 82.
14. Leeds School of Medicine Council Book 1, 8 July 1831.
15. Ibid, 26 July 1831.
16. Ibid, 30 July 1831.
17. Ordnance Survey, 5 feet to mile, 1850, Boro of Leeds, Sheet 11.
18. Leeds School of Medicine Council Book 1, 10 October 1831.
19. Ibid, 19 August 1831.
20. Ibid, 21 September 1831.
21. *Leeds Mercury*, 27 August 1831.
22. Leeds School of Medicine Council Book 1, October 1831.
23. Ibid, 10 October 1831.
24. Ibid, 22 October 1831.
25. *Leeds Mercury*, 15 October 1831.
26. Ibid, 29 October 1831.

CHAPTER THREE

The First Three Years

ONCE the School was opened, the need for formal Council meetings was diminished; it was sufficiently small for most decisions to be taken on the spot and be unrecorded. The Council met on only six further occasions before June 1832; in November to fix a composition fee of twenty guineas to cover all lectures and practical classes[1] and to arrange for the placing of a light at the entrance to the School yard;[2] in December Mr Garlick was to make enquiries respecting the supply of subjects for dissection and Mr Smith was to order a machine to illustrate midwifery lectures,[3] while in February a quart injecting syringe was purchased for £5, and £10 was expended on wax preparations for anatomy.[4] In May, to the regret of the Council, Mr Bell resigned and in July was replaced by Mr Carlin 'to superintend the dissections . . . to assist in procuring subjects and in making anatomical preparations and other illustrations of lectures — and to make himself generally useful in the School; Mr C. being expected to devote the whole of his time (Sundays excepted) to the general benefit of the school'. He was to be paid at a lower rate.than Mr Bell, sixty guineas for the year, but was allowed to attend the lectures.[5]

The Anatomy Act was passed in 1832 and the secretary was requested to write to Dr Somerville, the first Inspector of Anatomy, for information relative to the licences for practising anatomy. Applications for subjects were made to the Wakefield House of Correction and Lunatic Asylum and to various workhouses including those at Leeds, Bradford, Halifax, and York,[6] also later to those at Barwick, Holbeck and Hunslet and to Leeds Infirmary and House of Recovery.[7]

Dr Somerville made arrangements in October 1832 for the granting of the licence. He mentioned that the Anatomical Teachers in London had publicly renounced the practice of exhumation. It seemed that the local Workhouse Board in Leeds had reservations about the Act and he advised calm discussion and the use of every means to 'remove the objections that are so natural to those entrusted with the care of the poor'; he suggested 'removing the body to your premises for a few days only, say 3 or 4, . . . to demonstrate the viscera, returning it without disfigurement, paying the interment expenses and decency in the removal'. In November he wrote, 'I shall propose to the Secretary of State that he shall recommend your School to the Protection of the Legal Authorities in Leeds.' The situation was not improved when a month or so later in an attempt to make political capital, the supporters of Mr Sadler displayed a banner about the Anatomy Bill intended to excite prejudice against Mr Macauley for the part he had taken in its support and it was reported that some medical men of the town had joined the procession.[8]

As the end of the first year approached, a minor touchiness and jealousy of position came to the surface amongst the teachers, a question being raised as to the precedence in signing the certificates of attendance. Mr Thackrah stated that he had not understood that this was to be regulated by hospital appointments. Messrs Teale, Garlick and Hey conceded that as he was their senior they were quite willing to sign according to the date of their diploma and the matter was left to the 'private arrangements of individual teachers'.[9] When at the next meeting Dr Disney Thorp, jealous for his doctorate, objected to an arrangement which he conceived placed him below his proper rank Council had the good sense to remit the matter to the Sub-committee (Dr Williamson and Mr Thackrah) considering the Bye-laws of the Society[10] and it was eventually resolved 'that in signing any public document from the School, the names of members, not officers, shall be placed in alphabetical order'.[11]

Other bye-laws, which were agreed, concerned the equal share of each member in the property and responsibilities of the Society, covered the financial arrangements in any change of membership, the procedure in a vacancy — due notice, proxy voting and voting by ballot — 'two dissentient votes negative an election' and contained the following clause 'That should it appear at any time that the interests of the school are impaired by the incompetency or misconduct of any member of Council, such member shall by the unanimous vote of his colleagues be excluded.' Officers were to be elected annually, the president not to serve for two successive years. However, it was agreed that Dr Williamson be President, Mr Garlick Treasurer and Mr Teale Secretary until June 1834.[11] It is evident that the School was regarded as more important than any individual.

Some fifty years later, looking back to the days when his father was lecturer in these premises, Mr William Nicholson Price commented 'A few back rooms in the old Dispensary in North Street, which would hardly have compared favourably with the traditional two-pair-back of a London lodging, and a dissecting room, the ascent to which was difficult, and the descent dangerous, typical no doubt of the steepness of the path of knowledge, and of the peril which may result from slipping thereon, completed the local habitation of our good beginning. I remember well the little back yard in which the carriages of the professors awaited the conclusion of lectures.' But he corrected himself from the 'professors' to 'lecturers' and from 'carriages' to 'gigs' 'for they were less pretentious times'.[12]

Thackrah, who had suffered intermittently since the age of twenty-one from a disease of the mucous coat of the intestine, contracted a pulmonary infection and died on 23 April 1833 at the early age of thirty-eight. His major work *The Effects of Arts, Trades and Professions on Health and Longevity* had been published in 1832.[13] The Council paid £10 to his representatives as the estimated value of his share in the property of the Society.[14] His tenure had been short but he had none the less made a significant contribution to the first two years of the life of the School.

In the third year it was possible for students of the Leeds School to take the examinations at Apothecaries' Hall without any residence in London;[15] the prospectus was advertised additionally in Edinburgh; Mr John Hey became associated with the teaching of anatomy as well as of botany;[16] and £10 was set aside for prizes during the session.[17] There were still some difficulties in the supply of subjects. In August and September approaches were made to the Workhouse Board to request unclaimed bodies[18] and Dr Somerville wrote a tactful supporting letter. In this he explained the objects of the Anatomy Act: 'First, the prevention of Murder for the sake of the Victim's Body. Second, the prevention of the practice of Exhumation. Third, the affording an adequate supply of Bodies to the Schools of Anatomy without exciting the feelings of relatives and Friends.' He went on to show how successful the Bill had been in London, 'success as surprizing as it is gratifying: upwards of 500 Bodies have been appropriated to the Schools from the various Institutions in the Metropolis without the occurrence of any incident to give annoyance to Friends or even Inmates of these Institutions'. This success was attributed to enlightened views; that if the schools were once supplied, the associated crimes would cease. After only one year of operation of the Act Dr Somerville is able to say: 'The crime of Murder as connected with the supply of the Schools can no longer exist, and several murdered bodies which formerly would have been readily disposed of without a chance of detection, have from the want of this facility led to the discovery of the crime, neither is there any inducement for the practice of Exhumation, for as the cost of the bodies seldom exceeds £2 to the Students now, the Avocation of the Wretches, upon whom our professional education was formerly made to depend has entirely ceased.' The Act had had the same success in all provincial towns with the exception of Exeter and Leeds.

Dr Somerville pointed out to any Authorities concerned the strict regulations imposed by the Act which he must see were performed; 'I have always insisted on the employment of a respectable Undertaker who is held responsible for the interment of remains according to the Rites of our Church . . . as it is an important point to satisfy the Public mind that the remains are not treated with disrespect, I have always recommended that the funeral should be superior to that of the pauper and this will account to you for the sum of £2 which is paid to the Undertaker for this purpose.'[8]

Armed with copies of this letter members of Council 'waited upon' the Workhouse Board. The reaction of the Board is not recorded; it is however likely that the letter helped but inevitably delay occurred, so in October Dr Williamson and Mr J. Hey visited York to make enquiries at the Castle, Jail, Workhouse, and Hospital;[19] while the Magistrates meeting at Pontefract were persuaded in April 1834 to allow the use of bodies dying in the House of Correction at Wakefield.[20]

Skulls — complete, disarticulated and sectioned, male and female pelves and a wax model of the female perineum were purchased.[21] No doubt the latter region proved as difficult then as it does today.

It seems that members of Council were taking their attendance at its meetings less seriously, for on 8 February 1834 it was resolved 'that a fine of sixpence be paid by all members who were 10 minutes past the time and one shilling by those who are absent during the whole meeting'.[22]

Dr Williamson and Mr Wm. Hey were deputed to procure designs for a prize medal to be presented to each class[18] and chose a design executed by Mr Wyon of London. It was to be a 2 in medal with the head of Hunter as obverse and a laurel wreath with the inscription Schola

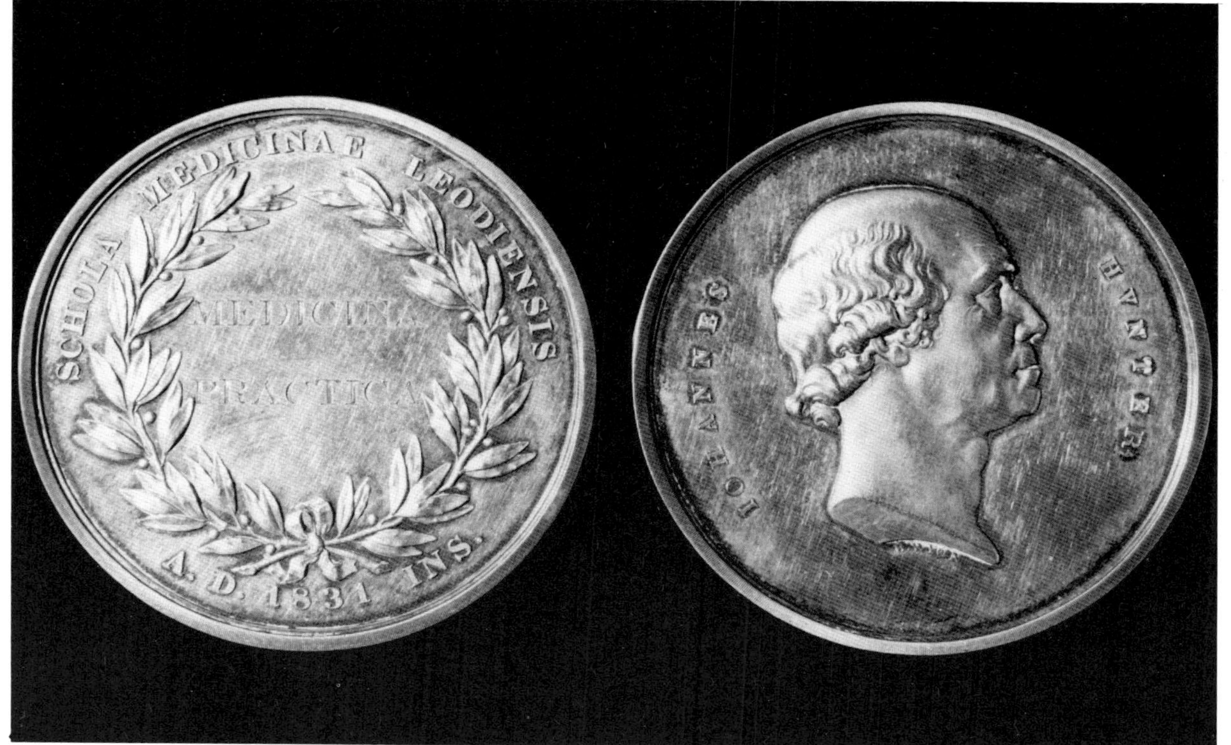

FIG. 5 *Medal awarded to H. Keyworth in 1834*

Medicinae Leodiensis AD 1831 for a reverse, the edge to be plain, not milled, so that the name of the recipient might be engraved thereon. In 1834 eight silver medals and ten bronze were struck.[23] Two examples of the silver medal, awarded to Mr H. Keyworth (Fig 5) are at present to be found in University Archives. A certificate of honour was also engraved, headed by the Leeds Arms.[23]

The Prize examinations were held in the first week of May daily, including Saturday, at 4 pm and the arrangements for them are interesting:

> 'That the time of examination may be prolonged to three hours to accommodate any pupil who may desire it.
> That pupils sign the paper containing their answers with some fictitious name, motto or device.
> That previously to the day of distribution of the prizes each pupil send to the teachers of the respective classes a note enveloped —the real name of the pupil being inserted in the note — the fictitious name, motto or device on the envelope. That the notes of successful candidates only will be opened, those of the unsuccessful will be burnt unopened.
> That one medal & one certificate of honour be given in each class unless there be fewer competitors than six in which case the medal only will be given.'[24]

The notes were opened and the prizes duly presented on Monday, 12 May and on the Wednesday the pupils entertained the teachers at Scarborough's Hotel.* The *Mercury* reported 'Nearly forty gentlemen sat down to an excellent dinner, Mr Charles Chadwick in the chair, Mr Graham acted as Vice Chairman. Several appropriate speeches were made, the utmost enthusiasm and good feeling prevailed and the evening altogether was spent in a very rational and gratifying manner.'[25]

The School was proving successful and viable. In the first year thirteen students had paid the fee to enable them to take all the courses offered and eighteen others had opted to pay separately for one or more courses, making a total of thirty-one students in all. The largest single class was in Chemistry, fifteen registered in Anatomy. Income from fees amounted to £301.2.0, which together with the £50 deposited by members of Council produced a credit balance at the end of the year of £23.9.6.

* In Bishopgate Street owned by Mr Henry Scarborough: now The Scarborough Hotel.

In the second year income from fees improved to £403 with more takers of individual courses. Bills paid included £2.11.0 for gas and £1.0.6 for candles. The credit balance at the end of the year was £121.0.1.

By the end of the third year the credit balance was £272.16.5. Certain small items of expenditure during this year are of interest — an ostrich was bought for ten guineas, a tigress for three guineas and a silver snuff box for two guineas. Income included £500 from fees, ten shillings from the sale of the tigress skin and a small amount of bank interest. In this session twenty-two students had paid the fee admitting them to all courses and the total number of students was probably between thirty and forty.[26]

Even in the School's second year the rooms at the Dispensary were proving insufficient and inconvenient and enquiries for another site closer to the Infirmary began in July 1833.[27] Later that month an offer of £500 was made for two lots of land in Park Lane (now the Headrow) near the top of Park Row[28] and in November £900 for land in South Parade.[29] An architect and a solicitor were appointed;[30] but neither deal proceeded, though a conveyance was prepared for the latter. In February 1834 it was decided to purchase premises in East Parade for £2000.[31] The site had a 50 ft frontage to East Parade and was 150 ft deep. In all these negotiations Dr Williamson acted for the School and indeed purchased the East Parade property 'as a private investment' from trustees who included Mr Wm Hey, transferring it to the ownership of the School by an indenture dated 1 October 1834.[32] In April it was decided to insure the building for £750 and in May the Council requested the Trustees to allow the School immediate occupation.[33]

REFERENCES

1. Leeds School of Medicine Council Book 1, 1 November 1831.
2. Ibid, 3 November 1831.
3. Ibid, 6 December 1831.
4. Ibid, 23 February 1832.
5. Ibid, 13 June 1832.
6. Ibid, 19 September 1832.
7. Ibid, 7 November 1832.
8. Correspondence taken from Volume MH74 — The Anatomy Letters Book 1832 — 1835 (Communication from H.M. Inspector of Anatomy).
9. Leeds School of Medicine Council Book 1, 22 September 1832.
10. Ibid, 8 October 1832.

11. Ibid, 23 November, 1832.
12. W. N. Price, *Introductory Address 1881*, Leeds Medical School Prospectuses 1864–84, p 7.
13. R. V. Taylor, *Biographia Leodiensis* London, 1865, pp 344–8.
14. Leeds School of Medicine Council Book 1, 5 July 1833.
15. Prospectus, 24 September 1833.
16. Leeds School of Medicine Council Book 1, 26 August 1833.
17. Ibid, 20 August 1833.
18. Ibid, 17 and 28 September 1833.
19. Ibid, 16 October 1833.
20. Ibid, 23 April 1834.
21. Ibid, 28 September 1833.
22. Ibid, 8 February 1834.
23. Ibid, 25 January 1834.
24. Ibid, 23 April 1834.
25. *Leeds Mercury*, 17 May 1834.
26. Leeds School of Medicine Treasurer's Accounts, vol 1.
27. Leeds School of Medicine Council Book 1, 15 July 1833.
28. Ibid, 25 July 1833.
29. Ibid, 2 November 1833.
30. Ibid, 13 November 1833.
31. Ibid, 12 February 1834.
32. Indenture, 1 October 1834. University of Leeds Archives.
33. Leeds School of Medicine Council Book 1, 22 May 1834.

CHAPTER FOUR

The East Parade School 1834–65

THE MEETING OF COUNCIL on 17 June 1834 was held in the new premises, No 1 East Parade, and Mr Garlick and Mr Hey were deputed to 'conduct the alterations in the building in conjunction with Mr Clark the architect'.[1]

Professor J. B. Hellier describes No 1 as an old substantially built Leeds house (Fig 6). There were four rooms downstairs, two of which were thrown into one to make a museum and the other two were used as lecture rooms or by the Curator. On the first floor alterations made a lecture theatre for about twenty-five students with seats arranged on the amphitheatre plan and also a chemical laboratory. Two attics were made into a dissecting room; skylights gave good lighting during the hours of daylight. A small dressing room was used as an injecting room for the cadavers, which were drawn up through a trap door.[2]

The dates of payment of the accounts suggest that the alterations took the greater part of a year to complete.[3] The costs of conveying the property and making the alterations amounted to rather over £800 made up as follows:

1834	15 August	Rawson	Solicitor	£50.0.0
	16 December	Woodhead	Joiner	£100.0.0
1835	28 March	Standish	Plumber	£142.0.0
		Barker	Plasterer	£39.14.0
	30 March	Woodhead	Joiner	£151.0.0
	2 April	Longley & Son	Bricklayer	£86.0.0
		Hogg	Mason	£49.0.0
	23 May	Singleton	Ironfounder	£77.3.6
	20 June	Clark	Architect	£50.0.0
		Rawson	Solicitor	£57.10.0

In February 1835 Miss Armitage who lived in the adjoining house, 2 East Parade, complained of an 'encroachment committed by the

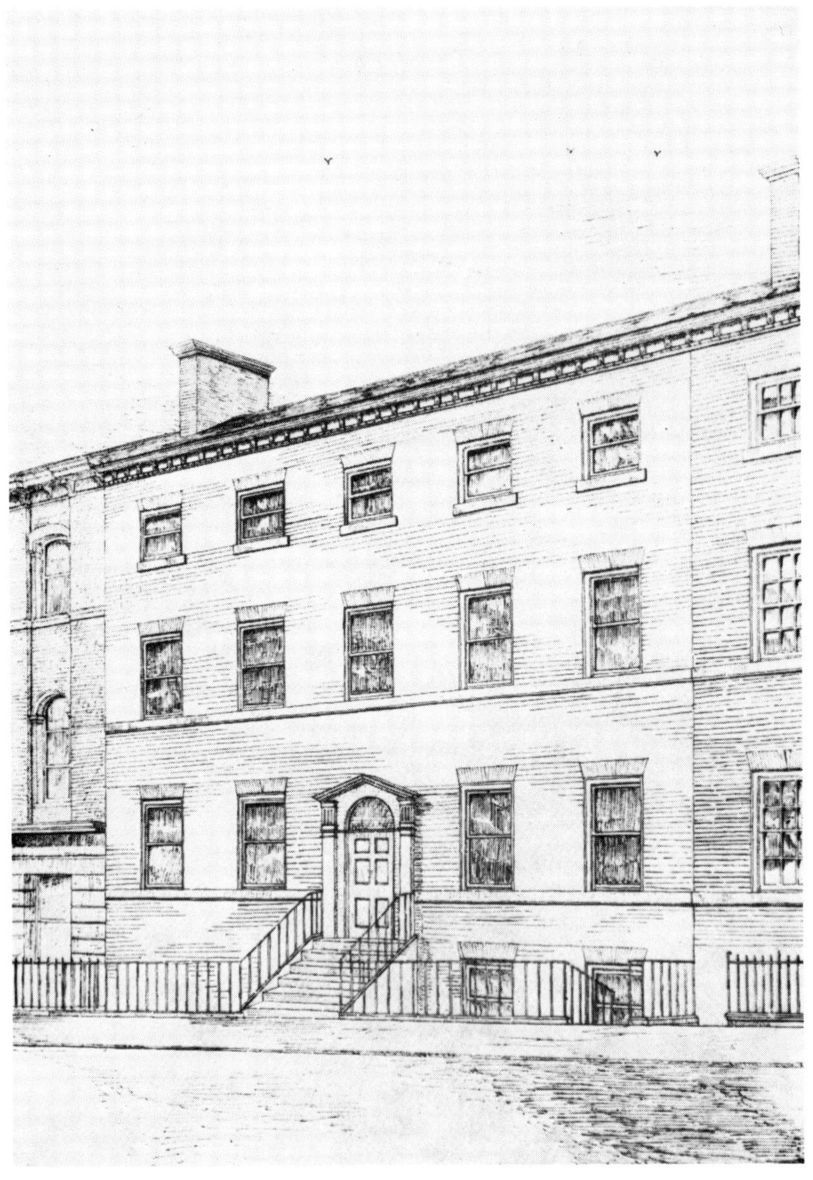

FIG. 6 *No 1 East Parade*

erection of an iron chimney'[4] and in March Mr Garlick was conferring with the architect about the alteration to be made to it.

It will be seen from the map overleaf that the new building was in close proximity to the Infirmary of those days — one minute's walk — and this was an enormous advantage. Mr Nicholson Price described East Parade as a strictly residential street and 'in order that the privacy of the neighbourhood might not be disturbed, for the property was held under very stringent conditions, no outward indications of the purposes to which the house was devoted were permitted. The students were obliged to enter and leave by a side door in St Paul's Street so as to prevent crowding about the front and other interference with foot passengers on the Parade.'[5]

The first session at East Parade commenced on 1 October 1834, under the presidency of Mr Samuel Smith, with an increased number of students, the vast majority of whom took tickets which admitted them to all classes. Mr Price asked for assistance with anatomical demonstrations and Mr Thomas Nunneley was appointed and became a member of Council. The income from fees increased to approximately £680 but the expenses were also greater, £90 interest on the mortgage being paid to Dr Williamson and the School now being liable for Poor's Rate, Water Rate, Lamp Rate and Highway Rate and of course for the insurance of the building and its maintenance. Despite Mr Nunneley's admission fee of £100 and rent from two outbuildings let half yearly at fifteen guineas and £5, the year ended with an overdraft of £36.15.7.[6]

After the distribution of Prizes, the pupils again entertained the lecturers to dinner at Scarborough's Hotel this time with Mr Samuel Hey, Junior, in the Chair and the *Leeds Mercury* again refers to the 'utmost enthusiasm and good feeling'. Perhaps not everyone was happy with the events of the day for the *Mercury* also printed a notice to correspondents:

> 'The letter of Justitiae Amicus containing remarks on the distribution of prizes at Leeds School of Medicine cannot be printed without a real name.'[7]

Such post-prizegiving dinners became annual events but in 1839 Council detecting a division amongst the students deemed it 'expedient to decline the invitations received from the respective parties' and instead invited the students to breakfast at Scarborough's Hotel at 9 am on the

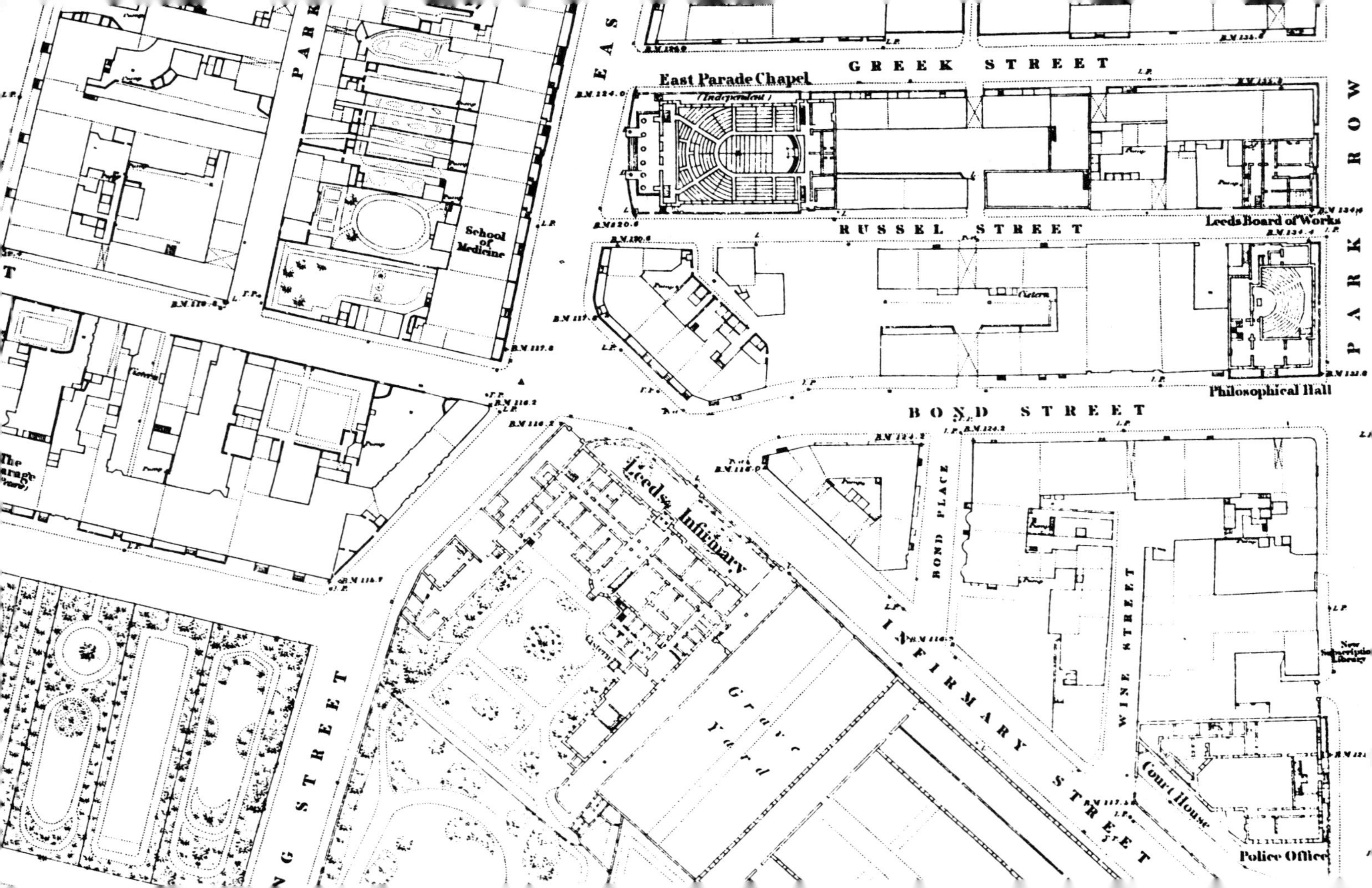
GREEK STREET
East Parade Chapel
(Independent)
RUSSEL STREET
Leeds Board of Works
PARK ROW
Philosophical Hall
BOND STREET
School of Medicine
PARK
Leeds Infirmary
BOND PLACE
WINE STREET
New Subscription Library
INFIRMARY STREET
Grave Yard
Court House
Police Office
STREET

morning of the prizegiving,[8] while in 1840 a Mr Langley returned his certificate in medicine in an insulting manner and Council decided not to attend the dinner if he be present and no apology received. Apparently he misbehaved again at the White Horse in the evening and was excluded from the School.[9] The following year Council agreed to the dinner if more than two-thirds of the students would attend. The time allowed for prize examinations was increased in 1837 to four hours, following a request from students.

The new building was more commodious and the Council now regularly met there instead of in private houses. Attention was soon given to the development of a library and to building up museums. A report was prepared in November 1835 to the subscribers to the Medical Library respecting its removal to the School, Council offering the requisite accommodation and in December the Leeds Medical Society was allowed 'the large room on the ground fioor for its meetings at 1½ guineas per annum for rent, fire and lighting and one guinea for the servant'.[10] Whether the library was transferred is not recorded.

In August 1836 it was agreed that a bookcase purchased by Dr Williamson be procured for the school and Council agreed in November 1837 to contribute equally with the students' society to the purchase of books, but in January 1838 decided to contribute £15 per year and students wishing to use the library would pay four shillings per year.

The purchase of books and the running of the Library was at first left in the hands of the Students' Medical Society but in December 1842 Council took over the management, following the exclusion from the Library of a student who had not joined the Students' Medical Society. In view of resolutions passed by the Society it was prevented from holding its meetings in the School for the remainder of the Session. Some students then refused to return books and Council gave up the attempt to get them back until the end of the Session 'when certificates will be refused to those people who retain them'.[11] By May it could be reported 'Nearly all the books are now returned'.

Dr Hunter's library of medical books was presented to the School in 1843 by Mrs Hunter. A compulsory subscription of £1 for all students was introduced in October 1858 and the museum could be used as a reading room from the end of the first lecture of the day to the beginning of the last. Some books might be taken home but new books used only in the Library.[12]

In order to build up the museum, members of Council in 1836 were encouraged to contribute to it by depositing their pathological specimens which would be regarded as on loan, their owners being free to remove them whenever they wished. Also Mr Garlick and Mr Nunneley went to London to purchase specimens and returned with upwards of 100. They included what might now be considered oddities — the femur of an ostrich, the crania of a turtle and of a crocodile and the vertebra of a shark. The nine foetal skeletons in glass cases however persist to this day in the Anatomy Museum. When Mr York retired as Curator in 1845 he reported that in the previous two years 138 pathological and eighty-one anatomical specimens had been added. Amongst the former were forty-four specimens of urinary calculi belonging to Mr Hey.

The fortunes of the school in the early years in East Parade were fairly evenly balanced. 1837–38 and 1838–39 were leaner years with fewer students and at the end of the latter year there was an overdraft at the bank of £35.15.0. The entrance fee of new members of Council could provide a boost to income for a particular year. In 1839–40 the number of students increased again and two new members of Council, Dr Pyemont Smith and Dr Chadwick, contributed £120 each. Dr Smith was the son of Mr S. Smith and both were former students of the school. In 1840–41 four new members of Council paid admission fees of £150 each and £500 of Dr Williamson's loan was repaid.[13] In 1841 the number of students dissecting in Leeds was 38, the second highest for the provincial schools (Manchester 50, Bristol 18, Liverpool 17, Newcastle 16, Hull 15, Sheffield 13, and York 10). These figures compared however with a total of 951 for London, where University College had the highest number (196), followed by Guy's (160) and Bart's (135).[14]

In July 1841 the School was able to pay the first dividend of £40 to each of the fourteen members of Council. Further dividends, usually for much smaller amounts, were then paid annually except in 1845 and in 1847–50, when no payments were made. Larger dividends were more common after 1860.[15]

Consider the case of Mr Samuel Smith the longest serving founder member who, when he retired in 1867, had received £360 in dividends over the years and a retirement fee of £84. This might seem a good return on the initial investment of £5 but seems less so when one considers that he had lectured in the midwifery courses for thirty-five years, twice weekly and at 7 am for no other reward than the honour. Others who retired earlier were less fortunate.

The School, in common with other provincial schools, was sensitive to factors which might threaten its existence. For example the requirement of the Royal College of Surgeons in 1836 that lecturers in Anatomy in Provincial Schools should undergo an examination before being recognised was regarded as discriminatory and the College was persuaded to rescind it in 1841. Mr Nunneley had been caught by this regulation and had needed to take an examination on changing in 1837 from demonstrating anatomy to the giving of lectures. In 1848 lecturers at Bristol had enquired of the College of Surgeons as to the meaning of a Bye-law concerning the Fellowship and on learning that this could not be obtained without attending three years in London at a Hospital or School, alerted the Lecturers at Leeds to the situation. Leeds agreed to co-operate in attempting to remove 'the obnoxious clause', and it was also raised at the annual meeting of the Provincial Association.

In February 1836 a memorial was drawn up for presentation to the Chancellor of the Exchequer 'relative to the claims of provincial schools being fairly considered in the arrangements now in progress in reference to a metropolitan University'[16] and Dr Williamson and Mr Teale waited upon the Chancellor to deliver it. Leeds recommended to Manchester and Birmingham that they do the same. An unsuccessful attempt was made the following month to obtain Royal Patronage for the Leeds School. In common with Bristol the Leeds School in 1845 memorialised the Secretary of State for the Home Office concerning an alteration in Clause 22 of the Bill before Parliament which would preclude graduation in medicine without two years residence at a university or medical school and requesting deletion of the words 'within 5 miles of Somerset House'.[17] In 1846 Dr Chadwick in particular was concerned at the effect which the proximity of the proposed Central Station would have on the value of the School property.[18] Such fears proved groundless.

After the establishment of the University of London the Leeds School in June 1839 applied to the Senate for recognition of lectures delivered at the Leeds School of Medicine and indicated such recognition in the programme for the next and subsequent sessions, but in June 1841 sent a memorial to the University of London 'in favour of such changes of the times of examinations as shall cause them no longer to interfere with the courses of this School'.[19] Degrees of the University of London were taken more frequently after 1858.

The first trial of ether anaesthesia in Leeds took place in the dissecting room in East Parade. Claudius Galen Wheelhouse, a student at the time, describes it as follows:

> 'In the dissecting room so far as Leeds was concerned, the principles of anaesthesia were born and developed. The wonderful news was brought out during my first winter session — that of 1846–7, that an American dentist, Mr Morton, has discovered that by inhalation of the vapour Sulphuric Aether, he could render his patients so insensible to pain, that without their knowledge he could extract teeth and perform other painful operations without their so much as knowing that anything had been done to them! Here was a field for experiment! We soon rigged up a large glass vase, like a tea urn, filled it with sponges, attached an india rubber tube to the spout, saturated the sponges with aether and through the tube inhaled the vapour as through a Turkish hookah pipe, and we fell over one after another quite insensible and unconscious of anything that was done to us. I well remember how I, as an early volunteer to take it, was nearly suffocated in the attempt. Indeed how nearly we killed ourselves or each other we neither knew nor cared! Here was a demonstrated fact, and from the dissecting room at the school to the operating theatre over the way, the fact was speedily conveyed, and before many days we saw patients operated on in this insensible condition and we found that they recovered quite as well as those who had borne the agony of the operation.'[2]

A surplus of cadavers occurred in 1840 and Mr Nunneley offered to provide a course in operative surgery, and again in 1847 when a letter of invitation to dissection was sent to all regular practitioners in Leeds offering them 'the usual privilege by the purchase of parts on school terms'.[20]

The Plan of Lectures for the fifteenth session in 1845 (Fig 8) shows the cost of individual courses and the number of lectures given. A new curriculum was laid down by the Society of Apothecaries for students starting on or after 1 October 1849 which would extend over a minimum of three winter sessions and two summer sessions. It specified the length of the sessions and the order in which subjects were to be studied; no surgery was included. The Royal College of Surgeons also issued a new curriculum but allowed the number of lectures to be at the discretion of the teacher. The Prospectus for the following year took account of the

LEEDS SCHOOL OF MEDICINE.

FIFTEENTH SESSION, 1845-6.

PLAN OF LECTURES.

THE SESSION WILL COMMENCE ON WEDNESDAY, OCTOBER 1st, 1845,

WHEN

WILLIAM HEY, ESQ., PRESIDENT FOR THE ENSUING YEAR, WILL DELIVER THE INTRODUCTORY LECTURE,

AT TWELVE O'CLOCK.

Course	Days	FIRST SEASON.	SECOND SEASON. Entitled to Perpetual Attendance. £. s. d.
ANATOMY, PHYSIOLOGY, and PATHOLOGY, by Mr. T. P. TEALE, F.L.S., Mr. NUNNELEY, Mr. IKIN, and Mr. S. HEY. The FIRST LECTURE, Thursday, October 2nd, at Twelve.	Five Days in the Week, at Twelve o'Clock.	140 Lectures. £. s. d. 6 6 0	4 4 0
DESCRIPTIVE ANATOMY, by Mr. PRICE, Mr. RADCLIFFE, and Mr. STANILAND. The FIRST LECTURE, Friday, October 3rd, at Ten A.M.	Monday, Tuesday, Thursday, and Friday, at Ten A.M.	100 Demonstrations. 4 4 0	3 3 0
PRINCIPLES and PRACTICE of SURGERY, by Mr. HEY and Mr. GARLICK. The FIRST LECTURE, Thursday, October 2nd, at a ¼ before 7 P.M.	Tuesday & Thursday, at ¼ before Seven P.M., & Saturday, at Ten A.M.	70 Lectures. 3 3 0	2 2 0
MATERIA MEDICA and THERAPEUTICS, by Dr. PYEMONT SMITH, and Dr. HEATON. The FIRST LECTURE, Wednesday, October 1st, at Five P.M.	Monday, Tuesday, Wednesday, and Thursday, at Five P.M.	100 Lectures. 5 5 0	3 3 0
CHEMISTRY, by Mr. MORLEY and Mr. WEST. The FIRST LECTURE, Wednesday, October 1st, at Eight P.M.	Monday, Tuesday, Wednesday, and Thursday, at Eight P.M.	100 Lectures. 4 4 0	3 3 0
PRINCIPLES and PRACTICE of PHYSIC, by Dr. CHADWICK. The FIRST LECTURE, Wednesday, October 1st, at Four P.M.	Monday, Tuesday, Wednesday, and Thursday, at Four P.M.	100 Lectures. 5 5 0	3 3 0
MIDWIFERY and DISEASES of WOMEN and CHILDREN, by Mr. SMITH and Mr. BRAITHWAITE. The FIRST LECTURE, Thursday, October 2nd, at Seven A.M.	Daily at Seven A.M.	70 Lectures. 3 3 0	2 2 0
FORENSIC MEDICINE, by Dr. PYEMONT SMITH.	In the Summer Months.	50 Lectures. 2 12 6	1 11 6
BOTANY, by Dr. HEATON.	In the Summer Months.	50 Lectures. 2 12 6	1 11 6
OPERATIVE SURGERY.	In the Summer Months.		

PERPETUAL TO ALL THE COURSES.................... £42.

☞ Application for Tickets may be made to Mr. GARLICK, No. 21, Park-Row.

N.B. Attendance on the above Lectures will confer the same Qualification for Examination as is obtained in the Medical Schools of London. The Terms for Attendance on the Practice of the Infirmary, the House of Recovery, the Dispensary, and the Eye and Ear Infirmary, may be known on application to the Officers of those Institutions.

CLINICAL LECTURES will be given at the GENERAL INFIRMARY, on MEDICAL CASES, by Dr. HOPPER and Dr. CHADWICK ;

On SURGICAL CASES, at the GENERAL INFIRMARY, by Mr. SMITH, Mr HEY, and Mr. T. P. TEALE ;

On MEDICAL CASES, at the PUBLIC DISPENSARY, by Dr. HEATON ;

On OPTHALMIC and AURAL PRACTICE, at the EYE and EAR INFIRMARY, by Mr. NUNNELEY and Mr. BRAITHWAITE.

FIG. 8 *Plan of Lectures in Fifteenth Session 1845–46*

changes and the course in Midwifery which was transferred to the summer months was given twice in 1849–50. The number of lectures in the individual subjects in 1853–54 were: anatomy 120, demonstrations 104, physic 100, surgery 72, chemistry 101, midwifery 66, medical jurisprudence 46, materia medica 66, and botany 45.[21]

In October 1852 students requested that the dissecting room be opened on Saturday afternoons and Council resolved that it be open at all reasonable hours,[22] but the students' request in 1854 for gas to be introduced in the dissecting room was turned down as 'not beneficial to the students and injurious to the subjects'.[23]

Personalia

There had been many staff changes (see Appendix 1). Although most of the Council were relatively young men it was a time when illness and death took an earlier toll. Thackrah himself had noted that medical men were at greater risk than was the population at large.

In February 1837 Dr Disney Thorp resigned because of ill health after an argument with Council as to whether he could resign without permission. He became too ill to lecture but left Leeds, recovered and was alive more than thirty years later. In December 1837 Mr John Hey died and this was a great loss to both the School and the Philosophical and Literary Society. The following August, Dr Williamson, who had been Mayor in 1836, became ill and had wished to resign but agreed to stay on with Dr Hunter's assistance; however resignation came in December 1839 and before he left Leeds a dinner was arranged in his honour. He declined the £80 retiring fee offered to him saying that he had 'never contemplated in rendering my humble assistance to the school any pecuniary benefit'.[24] Council decided to purchase 'a piece of plate' to present to him. Dr Hunter's resignation followed in June 1842 and he died a year later. Many of those appointed after 1839 were former students of the school.

Mr Teale and Mr Garlick were ill in May 1843 and offered their resignation but recovered sufficiently to stay on for a further eight and ten years respectively. Mr Morley, Lecturer in Chemistry, took over from Mr Teale as Secretary in 1839 and Mr Nunneley as Registrar for the Society of Apothecaries, but Mr Garlick retained the Treasurership until he retired. Mr Teale was later elected FRS, his name perpetuated in Teale's

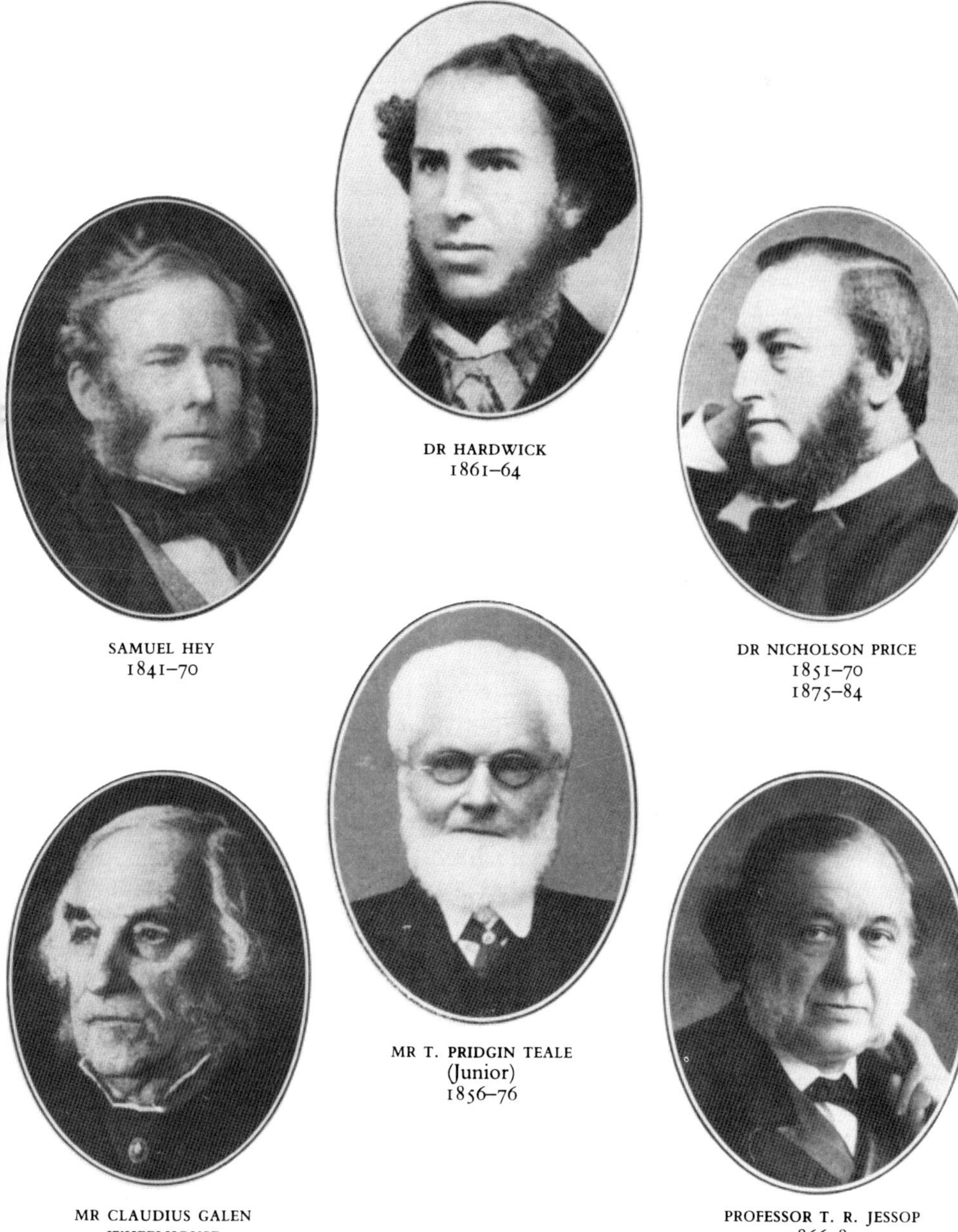

DR HARDWICK
1861–64

SAMUEL HEY
1841–70

DR NICHOLSON PRICE
1851–70
1875–84

MR T. PRIDGIN TEALE
(Junior)
1856–76

MR CLAUDIUS GALEN
WHEELHOUSE
1851–75

PROFESSOR T. R. JESSOP
1866–87

FIG. 9 *Some Members of Council of the East Parade School*

amputation. Mr Samuel Hey (Fig 9), son of Revd Samuel Hey and grandson of William Hey the first, followed Mr Garlick as Treasurer and continued so for the remainder of the time at East Parade. Mr Staniland, Dr Pyemont Smith (son of Samuel Smith), Mr Nicholson Price (son of William Price), Mr Wheelhouse, Dr Hardwick and Mr Edward Atkinson (grandson of William Hey the Second) acted as Secretaries during this period. Mr Wheelhouse (Fig 9) was a man of considerable presence and ponderous speech and is described by Dr J. B. Hellier as an able and graceful surgeon and a capital teacher.[2] Dr Robert George Hardwick (Fig 9), a handsome young man, whose name is perpetuated in the Hardwick Prize in Clinical Medicine, was born in Leeds, studied in the School and obtained high honours in the MB and MD examinations of the University of London. He became a member of Council of the School in 1861 at the early age of twenty-seven and very soon its Secretary; he was physician to the Infirmary, Dispensary and House of Recovery. He died suddenly on 19 January 1864 at the age of thirty.[25] The prize was endowed by public subscription.

Mr T. Pridgin Teale, Jr (Fig 9), son of the founder was appointed in 1856; besides lecturing in Anatomy and later in Surgery, he was interested in the ventilation of buildings and designed fireplaces, with sloping fireclay back and air entry below the grate, a number of which are still to be found in Leeds houses; they measure 15 in instead of the more usual 14 in or 16 in sizes.

Dr John Deakin Heaton who lived at Claremont, Clarendon Road, and who joined the Council in 1844, first lectured in Botany and then in Medicine. Mr Thomas Scattergood was appointed in 1851 and Dr Clifford Allbutt in 1864. These last three made greater contributions later in the life of the School and will be mentioned again.

Council was a powerful body, could be generous when generosity was deserved, as in giving the porter £1 and a week's leave to visit the Great Exhibition of 1851 — and to its own members in giving to their sons free tickets to lectures. It could be sympathetic in adverse circumstances as in paying the funeral expenses of a student who died and in paying £2 for medical comforts to Brown, the porter who in 1864 was 'suffering from abscess contracted in the performance of his duties', but could show plainly that it was in control if anyone stepped out of line, be it student, porter, assistant or even one of its own members. As examples, the following may be cited:

In 1844 Mr West complained of the disorderly conduct of two students — Batty and Hobden — and this was substantiated by Mr York, the Curator. They were called at 9 am for a severe reprimand by the President and 'Council deemed it its duty to make it known to their parents or guardians and on any repetition they will be expelled':[26] the replies of the parents were read at the next Council Meeting and copies preserved.

There were several cases of students engaging in illegal practice. In October 1844 Mr Settle was permitted to return as a student 'on condition that he pays his arrears, does not practice medicine during attendance at the School, takes down the board on his house announcing him a surgeon, that he shall be allowed simply his name on his street door, that he attend punctually'.[27] He obeyed the conditions. In 1846 the Secretary was authorised to enquire 'if the Mr Higgins who attends the Chemist's shop be the one mentioned in a handbill, and if he be he can not be allowed to attend the School and his fee be forthwith returned to him'.[28] In 1852 Mr Skelton was found to be in illegal practice with his father 'as an empirical practitioner' and further tickets (for lectures) were refused.[29] In January 1856 Mr Lodge was reported by the Bradford Medico-Ethical Society and found to be illegally practising in Bradford. He was required to take up his residence in Leeds (which he did) or provide a voucher indicating that he was assistant to a regularly qualified practitioner.[30] In March Mr Jas. Holt was reported to be practising in Castleford under an assumed name (? Mr Lewison of Rothwell);[31] his certificates were refused in the summer. When Mr Jepson the porter in 1846 applied for an increase in wage Council unanimously agreed 'that he is a most inefficient person and unless he improves he must expect to be dismissed'.

Concerning assistants: Mr Fielding, whose request in 1843 for permission to take charge of a practice for an indefinite period was refused and who then 'behaved to the Council in a manner exceedingly insolent and unaccountable and gave notice that he would leave the service of Council tomorrow' was dismissed immediately, 'with permission to return for his clothes and effects at an appointed time in the presence of two members of Council'.[32] In 1854 Mr Rayner, the Curator, was reprimanded and warned for irregular attendance, frequently having students smoking in his room and on several occasions staying out to a very late hour; the secretary wrote a private letter to the brother of the Curator stating the circumstances.[33] Council decreed that 'no smoking be allowed *anywhere* on the premises of the School'.

Concerning members of Council: When Dr Chadwick declined to accept the office of President in 1862 it was because he considered that another member of Council was acting unprofessionally; it

> transpired that a chemist, Mr Toulson, was advertising a testimonial given to him by Dr William Braithwaite and his son, Dr James Braithwaite, and said to be worth £7 per week to the chemist. A circular had also been printed from William and James Braithwaite indicating that they had recently taken their degrees as Physicians 'but this will not alter the mode of conducting family practice, neither shall we make any increase in our charges'.
> Dr Braithwaite who had been a member of Council for 21 years, declined to attend a Council Meeting when summoned, regarded the Council as exceeding it functions and finally resigned.[34]

The Queen's Visit

A significant event in the town was Queen Victoria's visit to open the Town Hall in 1858. The exterior of the School was redecorated and a calculation was made of the number of persons the windows of the School would accommodate to see the Queen as she passed along East Parade. It was decided that each member of Council requiring them could be given six tickets; places were also reserved for the porter and his family.

Overcrowding at East Parade

The class lists of the 1840s and 1850s showed the number of students attending the school to vary between twenty-six and forty-three. Following the student's name in the list there was a column for each subject, in which abbreviations were 'v.d.' or 'v.dil.' [meaning very diligent] 'v.reg.' or merely 'att', 'susp' [meaning certificate suspended] and 'ref' [meaning certificate refused]. Of the forty-three names in the 1844–45 winter session class list twenty-eight were satisfacory in all subjects and five in none.

In the winter of 1859–60 the number of students enrolled reached forty nine and it was necessary in the following summer to use the dissecting room for practical chemistry. Even more students entered in the winter session 1860–61, a total of 62, of whom 40 were studying Anatomy, 40 Physiology, 23 Chemistry, 25 Physics, 34 Surgery and overcrowding was worse. A Sub-committee consisting of Mr Scattergood, Mr Wheelhouse, Mr Teale and Dr Hardwick, was appointed in July 1863 to review the conditions and within a fortnight it produced a long and devastating report indicating that nearly every department was impaired for want of space and in summary listing particularly:

1. Chemistry: The chemical laboratory cannot possibly accommodate the students and the dissecting room has to be used. In consequence, dissections have to be carried on in the small private dissecting room, which is inadequate in size and hot in summer; also any bodies in excess of two must be stored on the floor in the materia medica museum, as the dissecting tables are in use for the chemistry class, and so cleanliness is difficult to maintain. A further disadvantage is that the room is not available to put up preparations and other work for the museum, when those willing to undertake such work will have most time at their disposal.
2. The Curator's bedroom is uninhabitable and he has no room he can call his own or occupy in case of sickness.
3. The library is too small and the shelves filled with books selected for immediate use. There is little room for additional shelves in consequence of one side being occupied by the Curator's bed.
4. The Anatomical Museum is over full and there is difficulty in exhibiting specimens and in getting at them; the floor is covered with specimens which are perishing from their dangerous position.

The Pathological and Materia Medica museums were more satisfactory save for lack of space (the latter had recently been completely refurbished by Mr Reynolds, Mr West's successor, of Harvey and Reynolds, at no cost to the School).

The Sub-committee strongly condemned the filthy state of the floors, shelves and jars under the care of the present porter and recommended that a new porter and a competent paid Curator, having no lectures to attend, be appointed, and 'to meet the longstanding defects there are only two ways open, either to enlarge our present building to a considerable extent or to be prepared to erect a new building near the future Infirmary'.[35]

Action followed quickly. Two weeks later on 30 July the advertisement for the Curator was agreed and in a further three weeks he had been appointed and suitable land for building had been found in Park Street. It had several advantages. It was near to the new Infirmary site, had the open space of the Rifle ground in front of it, which ensured it would not be overlooked; it was of ample size and had a convenient back street and also it could be obtained independently of the building committee of the new Infirmary.

A disadvantage was that 'a nuisance exists, an engine for crushing corn for Mr Peffer's stables, but this lies on the other side of Chariot Street' and the resolution to purchase was carried nem con on 28 August 1863 and was confirmed at an Extraordinary Council Meeting on 19 September. The cost was £1012.

On 30 January 1864 Mr Atkinson was appointed Secretary in place of Dr Hardwick who had died eleven days earlier, and it was decided to place the East Parade premises in the hands of Mr Hindle, the Estate Agent.

REFERENCES

1. Leeds School of Medicine, Council Book 2, 17 June 1834.
2. J. B. Hellier, *On the History of Medical Education in Leeds, An Address to Students*, 1921, Typescript, in Leeds Central Library.
3. Leeds School of Medicine, Treasurer's Book 1.
4. Leeds School of Medicine, Council Book 2, 13 February 1834.
5. W. Nicholson Price, *Introductory Address. Leeds School of Medicine. The Fifty-first Session* (1881) p 15, in Leeds School of Medicine Prospectuses, 1864–84, in Medical Library, University of Leeds.
6. Leeds School of Medicine, Treasurer's Book 1.
7. *Leeds Mercury*, 23 May 1835.
8. Leeds School of Medicine, Council Book 2, 6 April 1839.
9. Ibid, 7 and 16 May 1840.
10. Ibid, 22 December 1835.
11. Ibid, 6 April 1842.
12. Ibid, 30 October 1858.
13. Leeds School of Medicine, Treasurer's Book 1.
14. 'Anatomy Statistics of Students and Subjects 1842–1858' in Volume MH74 p 169, (Communication from H.M. Inspector of Anatomy).
15. Leeds School of Medicine, Treasurer's Books 1, 2 and 3.
16. Leeds School of Medicine, Council Book 2, 20 February 1836.
17. Leeds School of Medicine, Council Book 3, 3 June 1845.
18. Ibid, 1 October 1846.
19. Leeds School of Medicine, Council Book 2, 2 June 1841.
20. Leeds School of Medicine, Council Book 3, 14 May 1847.
21. Ibid, Class lists.
22. Ibid, 4 October 1852.
23. Ibid, 9 March 1854.
24. Leeds School of Medicine, Council Book 2, 25 January 1840.
25. R. V. Taylor, *Biographia Leodiensis*, London, 1865, p 515.
26. Leeds School of Medicine, Council Book 3, 20 January 1844.
27. Ibid, 28 October 1844.
28. Ibid, 24 February 1846.
29. Ibid, 24 April 1852.

30. Ibid, 14 January 1856.
31. Ibid, 19 March 1856.
32. Leeds School of Medicine, Council Book 2, 4 August 1843.
33. Leeds School of Medicine, Council Book 3, 21 December 1854.
34. Leeds School of Medicine, Council Book 4, 26 and 30 July and 5 and 8 August 1854.
35. Ibid, 17 July 1863.

CHAPTER FIVE

The Park Street School

THIS WAS NOT the earliest, but one of the earliest, purpose-built schools in the provinces. The architect was Mr George Corson, who also designed the Municipal Building, now housing Central Library and Museum, and also the Grand Theatre in Briggate. His plan for the new School was accepted on 27 February 1864, at an estimated cost of £2580 and he was asked to prepare detailed plans and specifications with speed.

In June an offer was received for the East Parade site, provided it could be purchased together with the adjacent site owned by Dr Heaton. The Penny Bank 'having already accepted Dr Heaton's Terms liberally ceded their claim' and the East Parade School was sold for £4500.[1]

On 27 July the Committee met to consider Mr Corson's finished plans but now the lowest estimate was £3334 and Mr Corson wrote 'The builders' tenders exceed my estimate principally in the Brick and Mason Work . . . I think the estimates are high but I see no chance of getting lower ones unless the whole thing could be postponed till October or November and even then it would be uncertain. There is so much work at present that the men will leave their work on the slightest fault being found with them. . . . In these circumstances the masters will not undertake work except at a price which will cover all contingencies and some will not tender at all. I am at a loss to see where a reduction can be made.'[2] Mr Corson was asked to readvertise, but when tenders were received ten days later they were £12 more than the previous ones.

The old School had been sold, the matter was urgent and Mr Corson was requested to commence the building, but revised plans, saving £419, omitted the tower and certain ornaments. The prospectus for 1864–65 shows a sketch of the school without a tower, but in November the tower was restored to the plans at a cost of £140. Ready money was required to pay contractors during the winter and Mr S. Hey loaned £500 in December and Mr S. Smith £100 in January, the loans being repaid with interest the following May.[3]

The old School had to be vacated in the spring of 1865 and lodging accommodation was needed for the Curator and the Porter and his family until the new school was ready. This was in time for the Summer Session 1865 which began in May. New trustees were appointed, Messrs Atkinson, Hall, W. N. Price, Seaton, T. P. Teale Jr, and Wheelhouse replacing Messrs Garlick, Wm Price, Samuel Smith, T. P. Teale Sr and Dr Thorp.[4]

Mr Reynolds had resigned and 'an opportunity for supplying Mr Reynolds' place in Chemistry was afforded by the arrival of Mr Fairley, recently appointed teacher of chemistry at Leeds Grammar School'.[5] He was to give two-thirds of the course of winter lectures and a summer course of practical chemistry. Mr Scattergood was to purchase a blowpipe table for the laboratory. Mr Thomas Nunneley complained that his name had been omitted from the Prospectus and resigned. It was explained that what he had seen was a proof sheet before amendment; he withdrew his complaint but adhered to his resignation. He had had thirty years' service and was elected an Honorary Member of Council but entered into an argument with Council when a retiring fee of £50 was offered to him. It may be that he had some right on his side, for five months later to avoid litigation £34 was added and he expressed himself satisfied. It set the standard for succeeding retiring fees.[6]

The Park Street building

The building in Park Street has a pleasing exterior (Fig 10) which can still be seen today, being presently and since 1926, occupied by Chas F. Thackray Ltd, surgical instrument manufacturers.

Standing in Park Street facing the front of the building one may note the main entrance, approached by a short flight of steps and deeply recessed under a gothic arch. Around the circular window above the two doors is the inscription SCHOLA MEDICINAE LEODIENSIS AD MDCCCLXV INSTITUTA AD MDCCCXXX' — curiously a mistaken date of institution, a year earlier than that given elsewhere (see pp 5, 26). The two windows to the left of the entrance belonged to the museum, a fine single-storey room, 40 ft square, to which a gallery was added in 1869. To the right of the entrance the first of the large windows belonged to the Curator's room and the other three to the library. On the 'principal floor', below the Curator's room was the Council room and

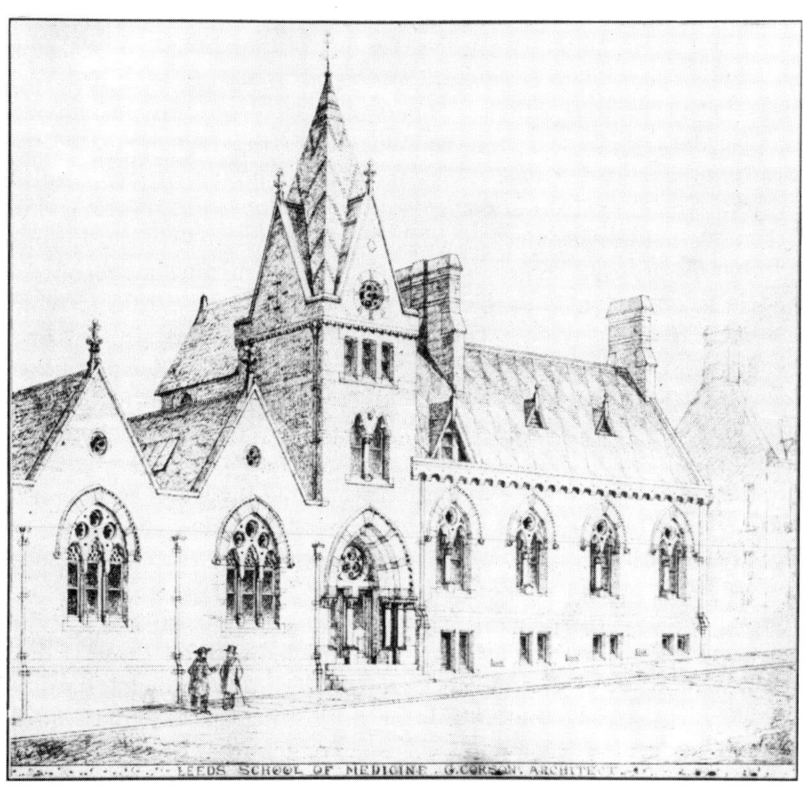

FIG. 10 *The Park Street School*

below the library were the materia medica room and the porter's rooms. The library had a vaulted and beamed roof. The frontage extends to 110 ft, the height to the eaves is 24 ft and to the finial on the tower 76 ft.

Those who have been into the building to purchase instruments will have climbed the short staircase to the library floor and passed through the door opposite into the sale room, which as will be seen from the plans (Fig 11) represents the upper part of the lecture theatre now floored in. The door they used was the student entrance to the back of the theatre. In this the tiers of seats descended to a central platform to which lecturers had access from the principal (lower) floor. The theatre was in fact central and communicated with the chemistry department on one side and the anatomy department on the other. The former contained a student laboratory 25 ft square, a private laboratory and a balance room and the latter a student dissecting room 20 ft × 40 ft, a private dissecting room and an injection room. There was a lavatory in each department.

The students' laboratory was 18 ft high, 'lighted by windows on three sides and by a skylight, is thoroughly ventilated through the roof and comfortably warmed in winter. There is sufficient space for twenty-eight or thirty students to work at one time and the tables are supplied with drawers and closet, gas, water, sinks and separate frames of reagents'. For general use there were large vapour closets 'for such operations as cause noxious fumes, large pneumatic troughs . . . Hoffmann's furnace, Black's furnace . . . air pump, balances . . .' The dissecting room had a glass roof for north light, good drainage and ventilation on the eaves and was warmed by a stove costing £3.15.0.

Some members of Council made personal contributions to the School: Mr Wheelhouse presented a tessellated pavement for the entrance hall; Mr Smith gave 'a valuable painting of a skeleton to be hung in the New Library'[7] and Mr Wm Hey paid £19.9.0 for the carving of the stonework of the porch.[8] Mr Thomas Nunneley, once his retirement fee had been amicably settled, offered 'to complete the stone carving of the Museum Windows as a presentation to the School' and further offered on behalf of his son, Mr John A. Nunneley, 'to carve the windows in the tower'.[9]

The Opening

The New School was formally opened on Tuesday 3 October 1865. The minutes state 'At 3.30 pm an Inaugural Lecture was delivered in the

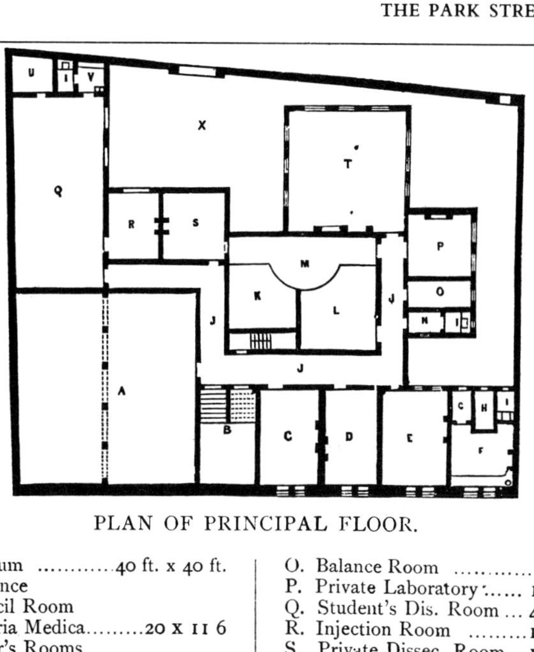

PLAN OF PRINCIPAL FLOOR.

A. Museum ....40 ft. x 40 ft.
B. Entrance
C. Council Room
D. Materia Medica.........20 x 11 6
E. Porter's Rooms
K. Heating Place
L. Store Room
M. Platform
N. Lavatory
O. Balance Room .... 6 x 14
P. Private Laboratory ...... 14 x 13
Q. Student's Dis. Room ... 40 x 20
R. Injection Room ....14 x 11
S. Private Dissec. Room...14 x 14
T. Students' Laboratory ...25 x 25
U. Macerating Room
V. Lavatory
X. Yard

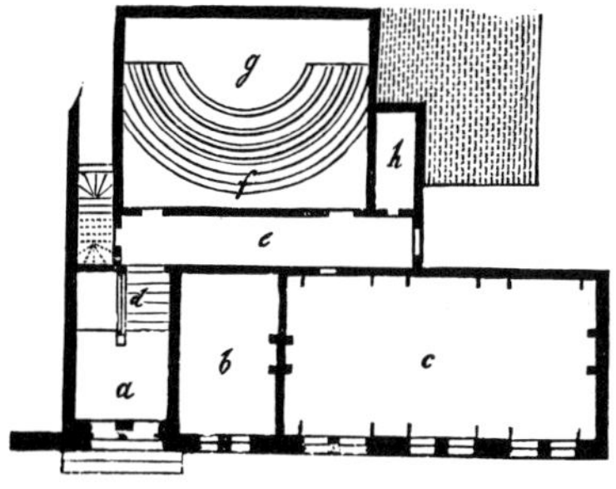

PLAN OF LIBRARY FLOOR.

a. Hall
b. Curator's Room
c. Library .... 40 x 20
d. Staircase
e. Corridor
f. Theatre ....32 x 24
g. Platform
h. Closet

FIG. 11 *Plans of the Park Street School*

Philosophical Hall by James Paget Esq. FRS before about 500 gentlemen including the President and Council of the School, the present students, very many former students from all parts of the country; a large number of members of the Profession in the Town and from the West Riding generally; the Mayor of Leeds and many of the Clergy and gentry of the Borough.'[10] Mr Paget spoke for an hour, somewhat eulogistically, but much of his advice remains as true today as when it was given. He spoke of the importance of acquiring the habit of accurate observation, of keeping full notes and reviewing them, of the educational value of examinations in general and of the viva in particular. 500 copies of his address were published by the Council. It was received with acclaim and two extracts are given in Appendix IV.

After the lecture the new Infirmary, then in course of construction, was visited and an Organ Performance was given in the Town Hall. 'At 6 o'clock all visitors from a distance were entertained at dinner by the members of Council at their own houses and at 8 o'clock a Soirée was given at the New School at which upwards of 200 gentlemen were received by the President.' There were demonstrations of surgical instruments by Weiss of London; trusses, supports and instruments invented by Mr Eagland of Leeds; new drugs lent by Harvey and Reynolds of Briggate; products of the distillation of oak by Hirst Brooke and Tomlinson; a cheap and accurate balance, Professor Graham's dialyser and a number of microscopes. Mr Samuel Hey, the President, referred to his own importance as he sat on the benches in 1831 to hear the very first lecture by Mr Teale, 'students being more desirable than lecturers'. He formally declared the school to be open. Mr Paget, having seen the Infirmary, professed his envy and said that unless they greatly marred it it would be the very best in Europe. Loud cheers were given for Mr Paget, for the President, for Mr Teale and for 'Old Sam' (Mr S. Smith).

'Mr Smith, who came forward after being repeatedly called upon, said it had been his good fortune to be one of the first founders of the school. (Cheers.) He was much obliged to them for the kind manner in which they had called upon 'Old Sam' — (loud laughter and cheers) — and he could only hope that in the course of time 'Young Sam'* would be entitled to the same kindness at their hands. (Hear and cheers.) During the whole course of his life he had entertained a strong love for his

* Samuel Hey.

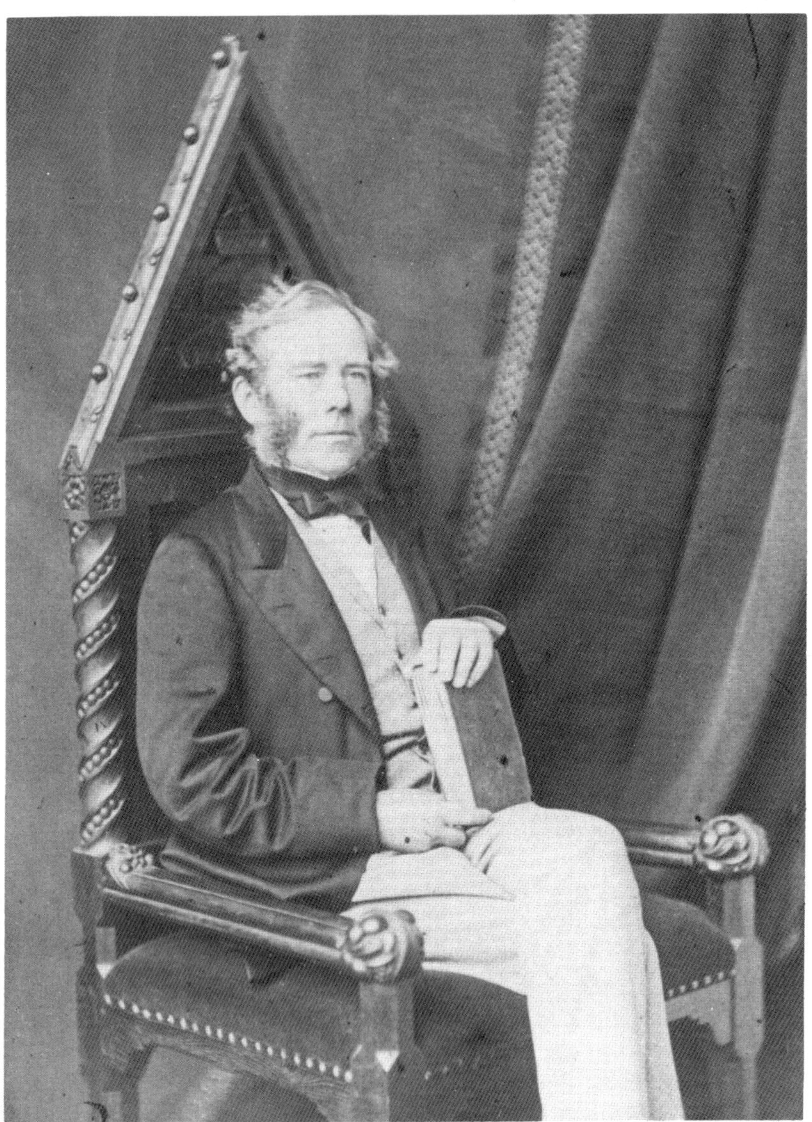

FIG. 12 *Mr Samuel Hey in the President's Chair, 1865*

profession; and, as a proof of that, he might state that, having now attained his seventy-fifth year, he was about to commence a new course of lectures — (loud cheers) — which he trusted would be productive of benefit to his students. (Cheers.)

'The company then partook of coffee and other refreshments, which had been furnished by Mr Powolny.'[11]

In Fig 12, Mr Samuel Hey is seen seated in the President's Chair. This was made for the Park Street School, has a carved back and arms and a red plush seat. The scroll on the upper triangular section of the back is inscribed 'SCHOLA MEDICINAE LEODIENSIS' while in the centre section of the back a shield is carved and around it, the inscription 'AD 1865' 'DEO ADIUVANTE'. In the Thoresby Place School the chair was used by the Vice-Chancellor for medical degree ceremonies which for many years were held in the Library. An iron clasp was then added to the chair to support the University Mace. The chair may now be seen in the ante-room to the medical Committee Room in the Worsley Building.

Samuel Hey was then aged fifty. At the age of sixteen he had been a student of the School in the first year of its existence, at which time he was a pupil of his uncle, William Hey the second. He was later at University College Hospital and St George's Hospital and joined the Council of the School in 1841, lecturing first in anatomy and then in surgery. He had just completed twelve years as Treasurer.

Much more space was now available in the new library. Dr Allbutt, who joined the Council in June 1864, became Librarian in November and he with Mr Scattergood and Mr Price formed a sub-committee to consider its management. Several gifts of books were received and in October 1865 the Infirmary Library was presented to the School. It was decided to advertise for a full-time Librarian and Mr Samuel Scott was appointed at a salary of £20 per year. The library was to be open from 10 am to 8 pm, every book taken out was to be registered, the maximum borrowing to be ten days, with a fine of one penny per day on overdue books.[12] Mr Scott's salary was soon raised to £40 per year on his promising to do secretarial work for the School.

The wages of Brown, the porter, were raised in September 1865 to £1 per week in consideration of his cooking the Curator's dinner, with 3/6 per week added for charring.[13]

In November 1865 the family of Joseph Prince Garlick, a founder of the School who had died on 6 June, gave in his memory a clock in a specially carved, turreted, wooden case, which for many years was in the Board Room and is at present in University Archives. Garlick had been Treasurer for the first twenty-two years retiring in 1853.

The Hardwick Clinical Prize of £10 for the best set of Reports on Medical cases was matched by the Surgeons' Clinical Prize, given by the Infirmary Surgeons. To these Dr Disney Thorp, the founder who lectured in Forensic Medicine in the 1830s now offered an annual prize in this subject, also of £10.[14]

The Infirmary

The new Infirmary in Great George Street (Fig 13) was designed by Gilbert Scott, RA, who was also architect of St Pancras Station, and neogothic similarities may be seen in the two buildings. Indeed Mr Corson adopted the same style for the Park Street School. Great care was taken over the design. Dr Chadwick and Mr Gilbert Scott visited the best hospitals in this country and abroad and the pavilion plan was chosen. It was to have 300 beds. The foundation stone was laid in March 1863 and the building was more or less complete in 1868. The total cost was £122,329 and in order to raise funds the National Exhibition of Works of Art was held in it for some months from May 1868. Unfortunately expenses almost matched costs and the Infirmary benefited only to the extent of £5. It opened as a hospital on 22 May 1869.[15]

With these two well equipped buildings the School could offer much to its future students.

Life in the new School

In March 1868, Dr Crichton Brown (Fig 14) offered to give six Lectures on mental diseases at the School and to hold a weekly clinic at the West Riding Lunatic Asylum at Wakefield, with provision of luncheon for the students, provided they were select and not too numerous.[16] In 1875 when he resigned having been appointed by the Lord Chancellor one of his Visitors of Lunatics he reported that average attendance in the last five years had been eighteen — the largest class of psychological medicine in the United Kingdom.

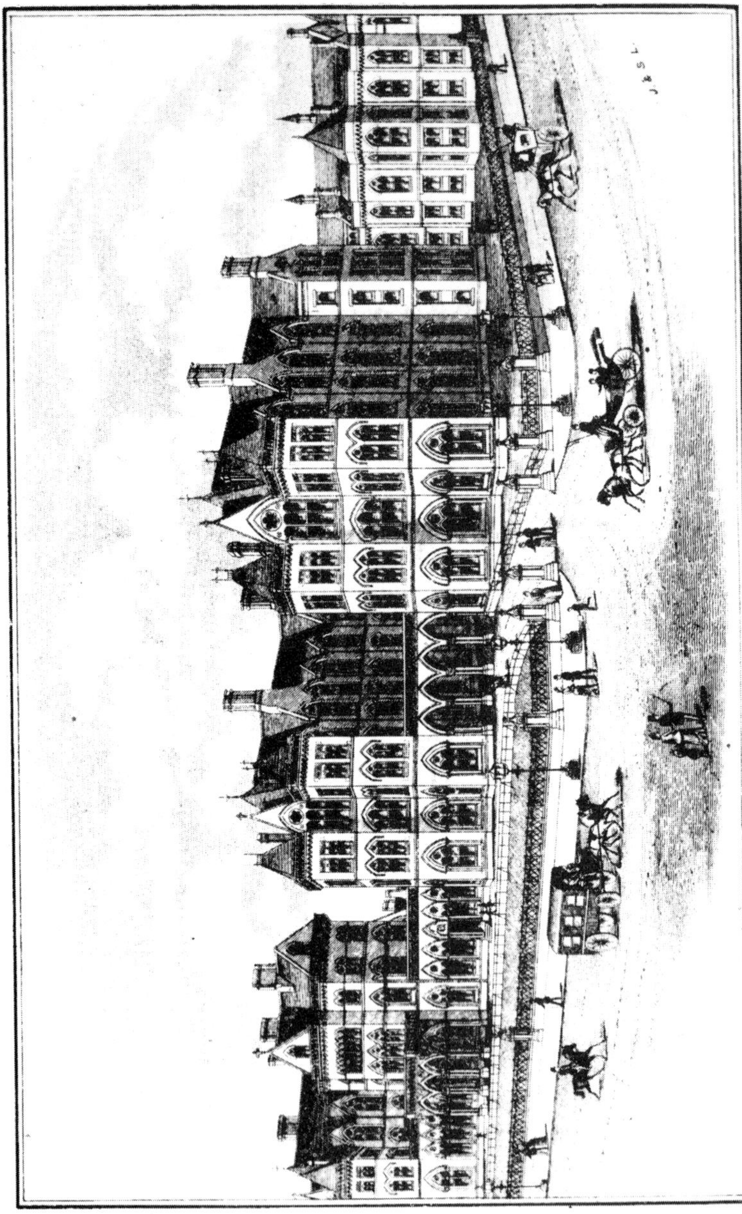

FIG. 13 *The General Infirmary at Leeds, completed 1869*

In 1868 consideration was given to making a second lecture theatre over the balance room and private laboratory at a cost of £60–£70, but it was 1875 before the decision to build was taken.

A course in Comparative Anatomy had been started in 1866 at Mr Wheelhouse's instigation to allow students to acquire certificates needed for taking the examination for the Fellowship of the Royal College of Surgeons. A separate medal given for Physiology from 1869 was a measure of the increasing importance of the subject and Mr Wright obtained permission in 1871 to expend £60 on microscopes, a further £20 on apparatus and materials. Professor J. B. Hellier, a student in 1871, describes his course as 'very defective in early subjects and in physiology'. The minutes of that year state 'The failure of so many Leeds students at the recent College of Surgeons Examination was discussed . . . eleven men had been plucked out of twenty-three and several of those that were sent back had been plucked before'.[17] As a result, teaching in the dissecting room was reorganised, attention was given to physiological chemistry and the 'great want of systematic teaching in pathology' was recognised in the appointment of Dr Eddison as Lecturer on Pathology.[18] There was no laboratory for practical physiology until in 1875 the chemistry laboratory became available for conversion on the transfer of the chemistry course to the Yorkshire College. The rise of laboratory medicine was beginning and Leeds and other provincial schools were trying to keep up.

In 1875 Mr Teale drew attention 'to the way in which the time during which students formerly dissected is now encroached upon by additional lectures and hospital work'.[19] The prospectus for 1865 had stated 'The supply of subjects for dissection continues to be steady and abundant' but in 1875 more were being sought and curiously it was John Brown, the porter, who was sent to see the master of the Tadcaster Workhouse.[20] He was successful.

Library

There was a significant development in the history of the library when in November 1874 the Medico-Chirurgical Society proposed the formation of a joint library and offered to pay £15 per year for the use of a new bookcase, it being understood that there would be mutual circulation of books. Mr McGill became Librarian in place of Dr Allbutt, Mr Jones the

Assistant Librarian received an additional 2/- per week for the extra duties and a gallery was added to the library at the cost of £100.[20] Numerous gifts of books occurred over the years, including a handsomely bound copy of *Cheseldon's Anatomy of Bones* presented by Dr Disney Thorp in commemoration of the opening of the 50th Session and a specially bound *Life of Dr Heaton* given by Mrs Heaton in 1884. For the warming of the library, the Treasurer in 1882 consulted Mr Teale and a 'stove similar to the one in Mr Teale's nursery' was installed, but Fletcher's gas heating stoves were used in the Physiological Laboratory.

Students

The number of students had increased and in 1880 Council recommended that students be allowed the exclusive use of the Council Room from 9 am to 7 pm and on Saturdays till 1 pm. Lecturers were to use the Materia Medica Room. The rule prohibiting smoking and assembling on the steps was to be adhered to. A further rule was posted prohibiting 'gambling and playing cards or any game (whether for money or not) in every part of the School premises'.[21] In January 1882 the Students' Debating Society was allowed to use the library for meetings.

Illegal practice by students appeared to be diminishing but other incidents occurred. Mr Gobal carved his name in new woodwork during one of Dr Heaton's lectures and was required to make it good.[22] Mr Thomas Sanctuary in a prize examination sent in answers of a very offensive nature and submitted no name. Afterwards he wrote to the Council that 'the papers were placed among the others by mistake and sent up by like mistake and that the whole affair was an entire mistake and misunderstanding on his part' and he apologised, but this did not prevent him from being forbidden to enter the School for the remainder of the Session.[23] Mr Johnson who let off fireworks in the school on 5 November 1878, was allowed back a fortnight later.

Staff

Much could be written about the staff of the School in the Park Street days for many were remarkable men. Sam Smith eventually retired in 1867 with thirty-seven years' service and his son Dr Pyemont Smith the following year with twenty-nine years. Their collections of calculi were given to the School and the old man's bust was placed in the library. Mr Samuel Hey retired in 1870, Dr Chadwick in 1871, Mr Seaton in 1874, Mr Wheelhouse in 1875 and Mr T. P. Teale Jr in 1876. The tribute to Mr Wheelhouse was glowing. 'His self denial and loyal devotion to the interests of the School, his great knowledge, admirable method of teaching and his strict punctuality have given his services a value rarely equalled, perhaps never surpassed in the history of the School.'[24]

50th Anniversary

Mr W. Nicholson Price (Fig 9) having retired was readmitted to Council in 1875 to help with the Midwifery Course. He was President in 1881 when the celebrations of the first half-century took place and gave the Opening Address. He was able to draw on personal experience for much of the history. He spoke of Dr Williamson and his contribution to civic life; of Dr Hunter; of Joseph Prince Garlick 'a more kindly and more genial soul there was not amongst us', whose teaching was plain and practical, who carefully tended the School in its early years and was full of good works in the world at large; of Morley, Smith and Thorp. He spoke of the extensions to the School built during the previous year (at a cost of £800) which doubled the accommodation in Anatomy, altered and enlarged the Physiology Department and of the more efficient warming of the whole of the School building. He examined the qualities needed in a medical student comparing some to those needed in an Alpine climber — physical powers, courage and self reliance, presence of mind, untiring energy, self denial, ready sympathy; he exhorted against procrastination quoting Sam Smith as saying that students invariably appreciated their opportunities 'long after the opportunity of utilizing them has passed away'; he advised that one should recognise one's limitations, 'take care you are fitted for the post you aspire to fill'.[25]

Afterwards the Annual Dinner was held at the Queens Hotel. Guests included the Principal of the Yorkshire College, Treasurer of the Infirmary, Chairman of the Dispensary, the Borough Coroner and the Stipendary Magistrate. The Mayor, the Leeds MPs, Sir Edward Baines, Dr Chadwick and Dr Disney Thorp had also been invited. Such larger dinners with invited guests had been annual events since being introduced by Dr Heaton in 1872.

REFERENCES

1. Leeds School of Medicine Council Book 4, 11 June 1864.
2. Ibid, 27 July 1864.
3. Leeds School of Medicine, Treasurer's Book 3.
4. Leeds School of Medicine Council Book 4, 8 May 1865.
5. Ibid, 21 February 1865.
6. Ibid, 16 December 1865.
7. Ibid, 21 February 1865.
8. Leeds School of Medicine, Treasurer's Book 3.
9. Leeds School of Medicine Council Book 4, 20 January 1866.
10. Ibid, 3 October 1865.
11. *Leeds Mercury*, 4 October 1865.
12. Leeds School of Medicine Council Book, 4, 14 October 1865.
13. Ibid, 7 September 1865.
14. Ibid, 9 November 1867.
15. S. T. Anning, *The General Infirmary at Leeds*, vol 1, Edinburgh and London, 1963, chapter 3.
16. Leeds School of Medicine Council Book 4, 16 March 1868.
17. Ibid, 25 May 1872.
18. Ibid, 22 June 1872.
19. Ibid, 30 January 1875.
20. Ibid, 30 January 1875.
21. Ibid, 10 June 1880.
22. Ibid, 17 February 1866.
23. Ibid, 4 April 1874.
24. Ibid, 17 July 1875.
25. W. N. Price, *Introductory Address 1881*, Leeds School of Medicine Prospectuses 1864–84 in Medical Library, University of Leeds.

CHAPTER SIX

The School and the Yorkshire College

ALTHOUGH a local University had first been suggested in 1826 by John Marshall, then President of the Philosophical and Literary Society, it was not until a trade depression of the 1860s that the superior education of workers in Europe was noted and real interest was aroused in the advantages that a College of Science could give to industry. James Kitson's suggestion for such a college was put to the Yorkshire Board of Education in 1869 and a founding committee was formed under the chairmanship of Lord Frederick Cavendish. The vice-chairman was Dr John Deakin Heaton (Fig 14) already a notable figure in the Medical School, who had been interested in education for some time and was to play a significant part in the early years of the College.[1]

Heaton was born in 1817, educated at Leeds Grammar School and became a student at the Leeds School of Medicine in 1835 while an apprentice of Mr William Braithwaite. After further education in Cambridge, London and Paris he returned to Leeds in 1843, being appointed Physician to the Dispensary. In 1844 he became a member of Council of the School and in 1849 Physician to the Infirmary.[2] He was President of the School in 1850, 1858 and 1872 and Treasurer from 1865 to 1879. His home was at Claremont, Clarendon Road, where he died on 29 March 1880.

By 1872 a scheme was ready for the College of Science and an appeal for £60,000 was launched. The first Leeds donor was Andrew Fairbairn, an industrialist, and to him and to Heaton was largely entrusted the task of raising the money, but it was Heaton who had to do most of the begging. By 1874 only one-third of the money had been raised, but through the good offices of the Nussey family, the Clothworkers' Company made a generous donation and on 30 April it was decided to go ahead on a revised plan and a constitution was adopted. All donors of £250 became members of the Board of Governors. Dr Heaton became the first Chairman of Council with Richard Reynolds, the chemist, and

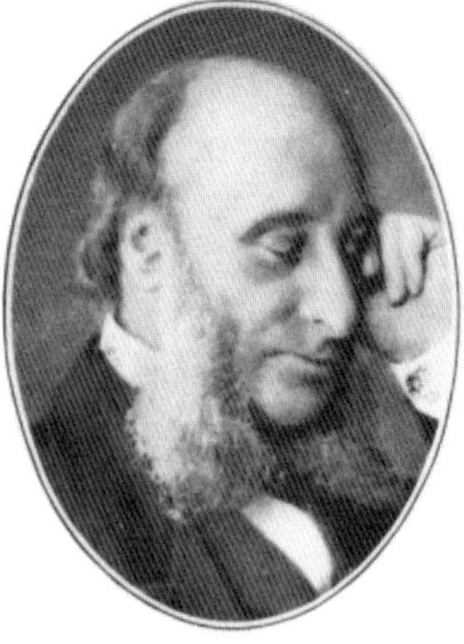

DR HEATON
First Chairman of the Yorkshire College of Science
1887

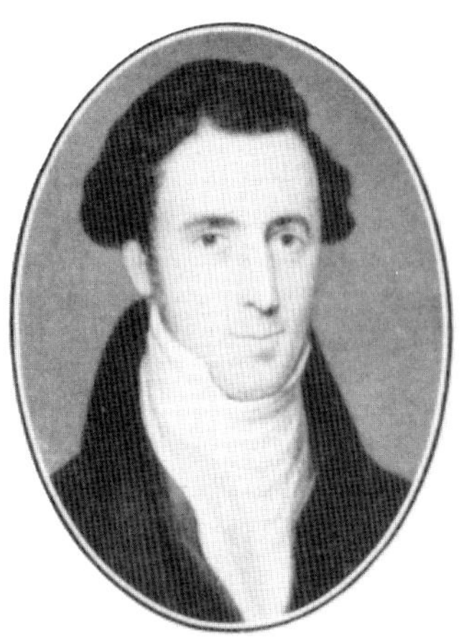

JAMES WILLIAMSON
First President of the Council of the School

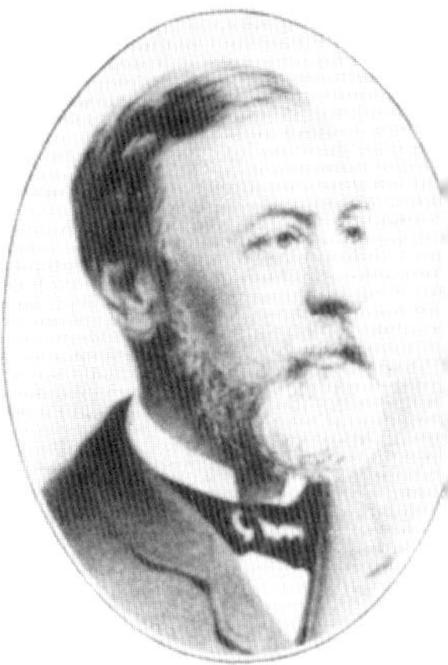

DR T. CLIFFORD ALLBUTT
Last President, 1884

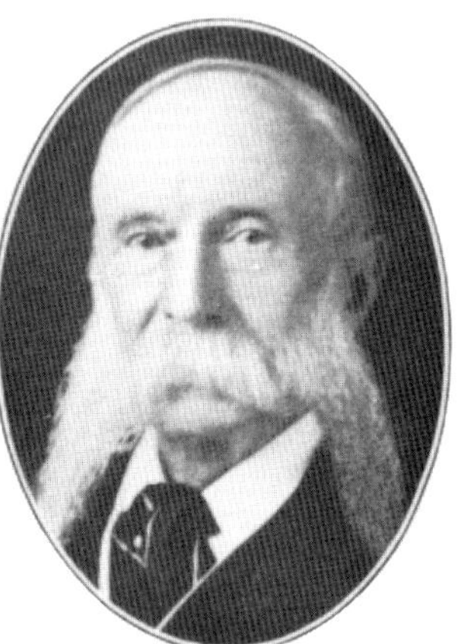

SIR JAMES CRICHTON BROWNE
1868–75

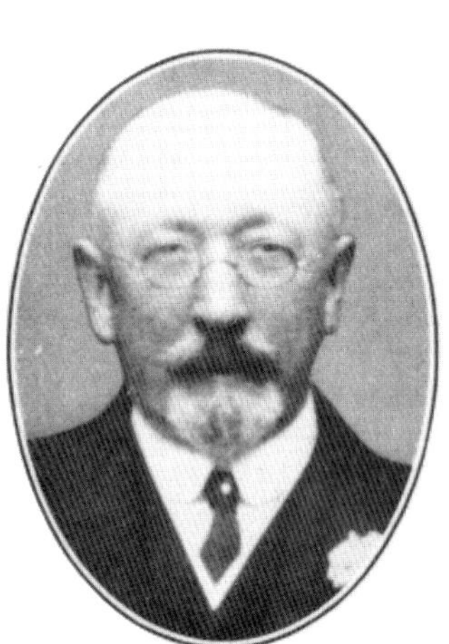

SIR ARTHUR W. MAYO ROBSON
1878–1909

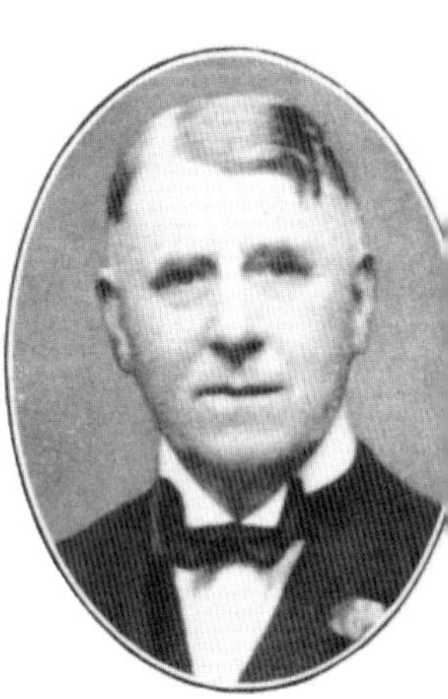

RT HON LORD MOYNIHAN OF LEEDS
1894–1927

FIG. 14 *Officers and three distinguished graduates*

Henry Sale of the Mechanics' Institute as joint Honorary Secretaries. The College was to promote the education of both sexes and deliver lectures in other towns in Yorkshire.

The Yorkshire College of Science opened quietly, without ceremony, on 26 October 1874, in rented premises, a disused bankruptcy court, in Cookridge Street, with three professors and one student. The professors were all to become eminent men: Professor Rucker who occupied the Chair of Physics later became Secretary of the Royal Society and Principal of London University; A. H. Green, Professor of Geology and Mining, was later elected FRS and became Professor of Geology at Oxford; Edward Thorpe, the Professor of Chemistry, was to go to the Chair at the Royal College of Science and was subsequently to be Director of Government Laboratories. They were joined in the second year by Louis Miall as Lecturer in Biology. He was Professor from 1876 to 1907 and was elected FRS in 1892. The number of students increased quickly, especially in extension lectures. Arts subjects: classics, modern literature and history were added in 1877 and the college in 1878 changed its name to the Yorkshire College, omitting the words 'of Science'.[3]

The Beech Grove estate was acquired in 1876–77 and the carriageway from Woodhouse Lane became known as College Road. The first building for the textile department was completed in 1880 but other departments remained in Cookridge Street till 1884.[3]

Transfer of Courses

In 1875 the teaching of chemistry was transferred from the School of Medicine to the Yorkshire College, but the School dictated the terms. College lecturers were to obtain the recognition of the various examining Boards; the dates of the Sessions were to be those observed by the School. The School would pay £2.12.6 for each student attending the winter course (four lectures per week) and £2.2.0 for each student attending the summer course (two practicals per week). College lecturers were not to sign Certificates of Attendance but were to report on attendance to the Council of the School.[4] Students were to continue to get their tickets from Dr Heaton in his capacity as Treasurer of the School. A list of the apparatus a student was expected to provide — test tubes, flasks, beaker, glass tubing, books of test paper, corks, etc — is printed in the Prospectus for 1877–78.[5]

Botany and Comparative Anatomy were transferred to the College in 1878, the latter course being held 'at the Philosophical Hall, the museum attached to which is extensive and well arranged'. Professor Miall who had studied anatomy and physiology at the School in 1867–69, was to give both courses.[5] In October 1882 the botanical museum was offered to the Yorkshire College, but in fact remained at the School until proper accommodation could be provided for it.[6]

Medical education had been changing. The Medical Act of 1858 set up the General Medical Council, which made recommendations, not at first binding, concerning the curriculum, but by 1869 the Prospectus quotes 'Every Medical Student shall be registered in the manner prescribed by the General Medical Council, but not until he has passed a Preliminary Examination as a test of general education' and a four-year organised curriculum was recommended. In the 1870s the apprenticeship was in great disfavour, nearly all students spending at least two years in hospital practice.[7]

The Yorkshire College was concerned in 1877 at the request of Owens College Manchester for University status.[3] In April 1878 the School supported a Yorkshire College petition to the Privy Council in favour of *recognising the claims of other institutions* in the charter of the proposed new University,[8] and a further Memorial in May 1879 'praying that a Charter to be granted for a new University (to be called the "Victoria University") having its seat in Manchester and suggesting a revised Constitution'.[9]

The Victoria University received its Charter in 1880 but the Yorkshire College had to wait until 1887 before being admitted as a constituent college, partly because its total curriculum was too technological and not sufficiently widely based.[3]

Union of School and College

The Yorkshire College in May 1883 invited the School to consider what action should be taken in regard to the Victoria University, which had recently been granted powers to confer degrees in Medicine.[10] A joint committee was formed and reported in August that they thought amalgamation between the School and the College desirable.[11]

Mr Scattergood suggested a form of offer to be made to the College and the President (Dr Allbutt) proposed 'The Council of the Medical

School will on the 1st August next hand over to the College the freehold land and buildings in Park Street . . . subject to the existing mortgages upon them amounting to £2500, with the fittings and furniture of the School, the Library, Museums and apparatus' on condition that the College pay the Council £2500, defray the legal costs and fulfil all contracts for the education of students. The School undertook to canvass for subscriptions to endow a Chair of Physiology and offered to head the list with £1000 provided the College would also take an active part in the canvass. The mode of carrying on the School was to be determined by the two bodies jointly.[11] The Yorkshire College accepted the offer on 21 September 1883 and appointed Mr Denison, Mr Lupton, Mr Reynolds, Principal Bodington, and Professor Thorpe to continue the negotiations.[12] Representatives on behalf of the School were Dr Churton, Mr Scattergood, Mr Wright, and Mr McGill.

Negotiations proceeded carefully and were ratified by legal agreement within the year. Each body needed the other. Provincial medical schools were finding it increasingly difficult on their own to provide courses which kept pace with the advances in basic science and indeed those schools which survived were all related to colleges of science. For a college the presence of an associated medical school was likely to hasten University status.

At one stage the School almost withdrew. It seemed that some businessmen on the Council of the College favoured technology and considered Arts and Science as of secondary importance. Dr Allbutt (Fig 14) on 7 February 1884 wrote to Sir Edward Baines that 'if such a view prevailed the prospect of joining the Victoria University would be indefinitely postponed. In such case the Medical School would derive no advantage from union which would compensate for the loss of independence and self governement'.[13]

The proposals which emerged for the governing of the College were essentially that there be two boards, one for the subjects taught at the College and one for Medicine, and that Medicine should have one-third of the seats on Senate.[14] After argument it was finally agreed that Senate should be represented on Council by Principal Bodington and one voting member elected by the Faculty of Medicine.[15]

On the financial side, the accounts of the Medical Department were to be kept separate, and after certain prior charges on the gross receipts the residue was to be divided amongst the professors and lecturers.

The prior changes were to cover the interest on the mortgage; make up the salary of the Professor of Physiology to £300; to provide capitation fees for the Professors of Chemistry and Botany and to the College for courses taken there; to provide the running expenses of the School, the salaries of the Dean and Demonstrators, secretarial expenses and a contribution to the Reserve Fund. The arrangements were to be reviewed in three years.[16]

For 1884–85 it was recommended that the Demonstrator in Anatomy receive £150, the Demonstrator in Chemistry £20, the Dean £25 and the College for secretarial expenses £25. Lecturers, with some exceptions, were to be paid from the residue according to the number of lectures each gave.[17]

Meantime in 1882 the possibility of starting a Dental course had been considered. Advice was taken from Mr Carter, Surgeon-Dentist to the Infirmary, the Royal College of Surgeons, the Secretary of the BDA and other schools having Dental Departments, Birmingham, Liverpool, Plymouth, and Exeter. It appeared that there would be no problems about lectures but the scheme was postponed because 'at present it would not be possible to provide sufficient facilities for practical chemistry'.[18] In October 1883 the School was to be connected to the Telephone Exchange, up to £10 being set aside for the purpose.[12]

At an extraordinary meeting of Council held on 16 July 1884, the President, Treasurer and Secretary were reappointed 'till the duties of the present Council cease', a dividend of £60 was paid to each member and the draft agreement for union with the Yorkshire College was approved unanimously and ratified three weeks later on 7 August 1884.[19] The first meeting of the Medical Department of the Yorkshire College was held on 6 August 1884 with Principal Bodington in the chair at which a House Committee was set up to care for the buildings and arrangements for a second porter made. Mr Scattergood was asked to be Dean,[20] a post which he agreed to accept on the condition that he receive no salary for the first year.

On 11 August, when the purchase money was received from the Yorkshire College, a further £132 per member was distributed, with an extra £25 for Dr Jacob 'in consideration of his having recently paid a higher entrance fee'. A cheque for £1000 was handed back to the College as the Council's subscription to the Physiological Endowment Fund.[21]

The only further meetings of the Council of the School were in the nature of tidying up operations. On 15 January 1885 the Treasurer presented the final accounts. Apart from £52.15.7 in the Prize funds there was a balance of

£70.19.3½. The sum of £70 was divided equally between the fourteen members of Council and the remainder after payments of any petty expenses 'given to the Charity Organisation Society'. Two further meetings in April and June 1887 were concerned with the transfer of Prize Fund Trusts to the Yorkshire College. Thus ended the independent phase of the School's existence.

Early years in the College

During the winter sessions of 1884 and 1885 special clinical lectures were given by retired members of staff: Dr Allbutt, Mr Wheelhouse and Mr Teale.[22]

Dr T. Clifford Allbutt (later Sir Clifford), who had retired at the time of the union with the College, was the most distinguished physician Leeds has possessed. Born in Dewsbury, educated at St Peter's School York, Cambridge, London, and Paris, he had been elected physician to the Infirmary and member of Council of the School in 1864. He invented the short-stemmed clinical thermometer and introduced the ophthalmoscope, weighing machine and microscope to the wards. He was described by George Eliot as a 'good, clever and graceful man, enough to enable one to be cheerful under the horrible smoke of ugly Leeds'. He was elected FRS, was later Regius Professor of Physic at Cambridge, and received no fewer than nine honorary degrees.

A students' Musical Society arose in autumn 1884, and had leave to use the library and 'place a piano in the Dean's Office'.[23]

Professors Eddison (Medicine), Jessop (Surgery), McGill (Anatomy), and Birch (Physiology) with Mr Scattergood (Dean) (Figs 15, 9, 15 and 16 respectively) had seats on Senate and Professor Eddison who had represented the School since 1878 on the Council of the College continued to do so.[24]

The effects of being part of a larger organisation were soon evident with an increase in bye-laws for the conduct of meetings and the development of committee structure. Cap and gown were worn for the Prince of Wales' visit in July 1885 to open the College buildings and for inaugural lectures.

The dissecting room remained open in the summer session of 1885 and a course of applied anatomy was given to the third and fourth years,[25] while in the following winter a course in advanced physiology was given

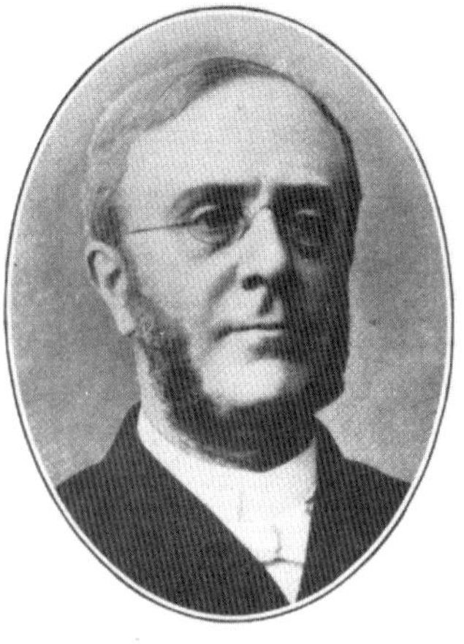

DR JAMES BRAITHWAITE
1875–89

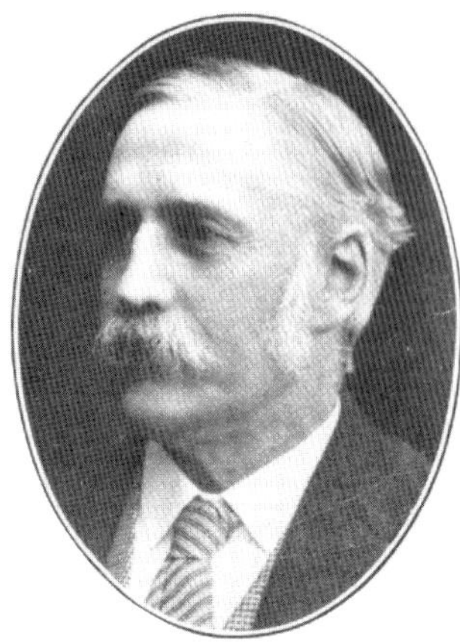

PROFESSOR J. E. EDDISON
1868–98

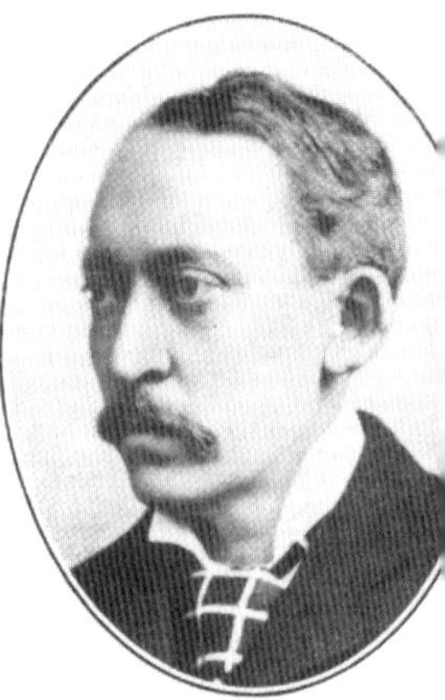

PROFESSOR A. F. McGILL
1875–90

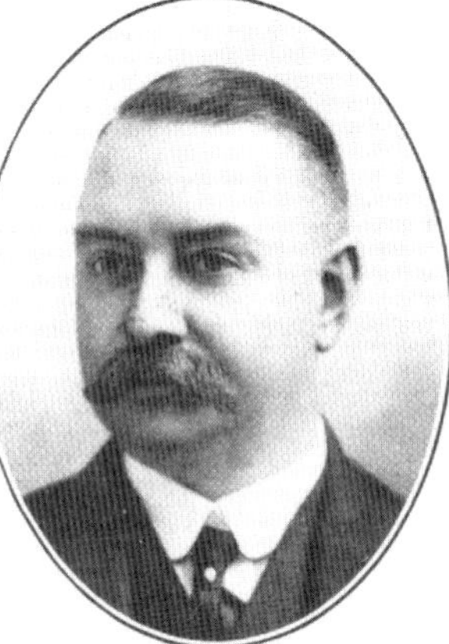

PROFESSOR H. LITTLEWOOD
1890–1910

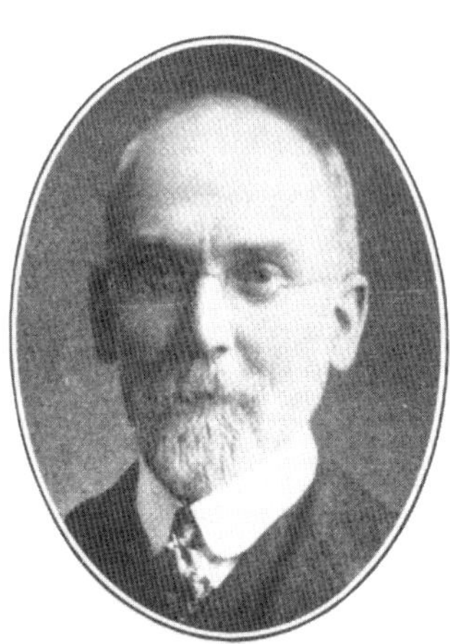

PROFESSOR EDWARD WARD
1884–1905

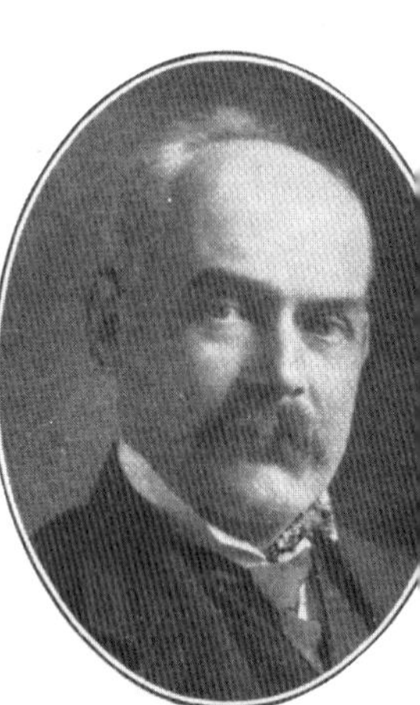

PROFESSOR E. F. TREVELYAN
1894–1904

for the seven students taking Primary FRCS or the London MB.[26] In January 1886 it was reported that the School was 'fully able to provide for the requirements for degrees of the Victoria University'.[27] However, in October 1886 there was concern at the number of students who were plucked in the first-year chemistry examination and were still carrying it in their third year. Professor Smithells (Chemistry) believed medical students did not take chemistry seriously 'being a subject long considered subsidiary and non-essential'.[28]

Victoria University

On 20 April 1887 the Yorkshire College applied for admission as a constituent College of the Victoria University and was admitted on 3 November.[29] Professor Jessop and Mr Edward Atkinson resigned in June to facilitate an 'entirely new arrangement of the Surgery Course'. Professor Jessop had served twenty-one years and Mr Atkinson twenty-five years (five years in anatomy, nine in botany and eleven in surgery).[30] During this period surgery was able to advance consequent on the use of anaesthesia and on Lister's work on antisepsis.

Thomas Richard Jessop, born at Brighouse and an old student of the School, was a man of massive intellect and 'grandeur of character unsurpassed'. In his examination of a case he was 'methodical, comprehensive and deliberate . . . nothing in . . . history or signs . . . escaped him'. He is credited with the first successful removal in this country of a tumour in the kidney and with being the safest operator on the staff; he was imperturbable. He remained in general practice and saw as many medical as surgical cases. In 1901 he was a vice-president of the Royal College of Surgeons,[31] a rare distinction for one from the provinces.

On these resignations Professor A. F. McGill transferred from the Chair of Anatomy to the Chair of Surgery. Three months earlier, on 24 March 1887, he had become the first surgeon ever to perform a suprapubic prostatectomy. Moynihan was his dresser acting as his house-surgeon and relates that a tumour, a projecting mass near the internal meatus was removed, which proved on sectioning to be prostate. When told McGill said 'Oh, was it, then why don't we always take the prostate out?' and at the BMA meeting in Leeds two years later he showed a number of patients, a row of old men, each holding his prostate in a jar.[31] McGill suffered from diabetes and died in 1890 at the early age of forty-four. His desk is still to be seen in the Consultants' Room at the entrance to the Infirmary. Mr Arthur Mayo Robson, later Sir Arthur (Fig 14) transferred with McGill from Anatomy to be Lecturer in Surgery and succeeded him as Professor in 1890 after only three years. T. Wardrop Griffith followed McGill as Professor of Anatomy and was himself to transfer in 1910 to the Chair of Medicine. In passing one may note the greater ease and frequency of transfer between disciplines which prevailed in those days.[32]

In June 1888 Mr Scattergood (Fig 16) resigned his lectureship in Forensic Medicine after thirty-seven years in the School, but was persuaded to retain the Office of Dean — an office to which he was re-elected annually and unopposed for the next eleven years and which he held till his death in February 1900.[33]

In the first decade in the Yorkshire College changes in the curriculum occurred. From 1886 botany was no longer required for the examinations of the Royal Colleges but the following year physics was needed by the Victoria University. In 1888 there was much discussion about holding Conjoint Board examinations at local centres but local colleges could not agree on where they should be. On 11 December 1884 students petitioned (successfully) for the continuation of a test examination in anatomy.[34] In 1891 a pre-registration year of chemistry, physics and biology was advocated and by the end of the decade a five-year curriculum was in being.

Occasional disturbances in lectures were reported, the making of noises and the throwing of pellets and comfits in one of Mr Atkinson's lectures in 1885 and the letting off of an explosive device containing gunpowder in one of Dr Hellier's November lectures in 1893. Twice the students' common room was closed because of breakage of furniture. When it was reopened in 1887 after a closure of ten months a letter signed by 110 students thanked the Board for refurnishing it and requested permission to smoke there. How much smoke was expected can only be guessed, but the Board granting permission to smoke after 12 noon, agreed that 'if found desirable a chimney breast ventilator be placed in the wall of the room near the ceiling and that the windows be adapted for convenience of ventilation'.[35] There was to be no smoking on the steps or elsewhere in the building.

The library received many gifts, Dr Allbutt being particularly generous. Books which had been stored in the tower were moved to the

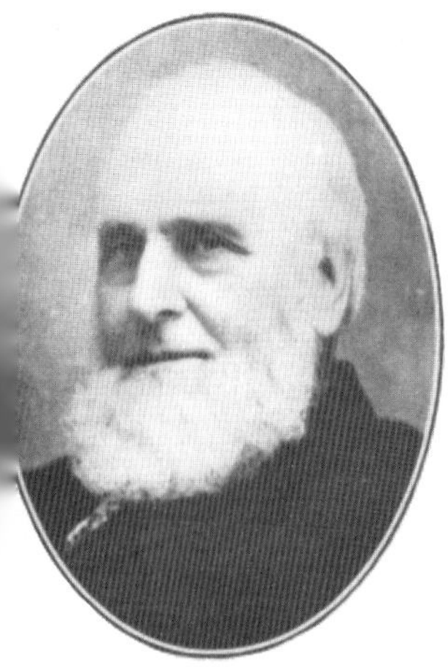

THOMAS SCATTERGOOD
irst Dean of the Department of
Medicine, Yorkshire College
1884–1900

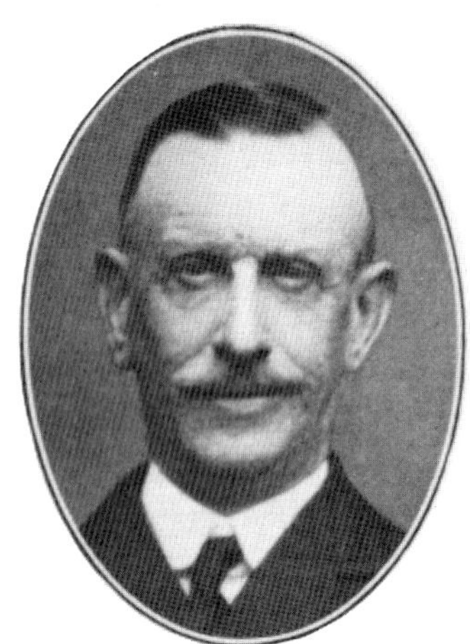

PROFESSOR DE BURGH BIRCH
First Dean of the Faculty of Medicine
University of Leeds
1900–06 and 1913–17

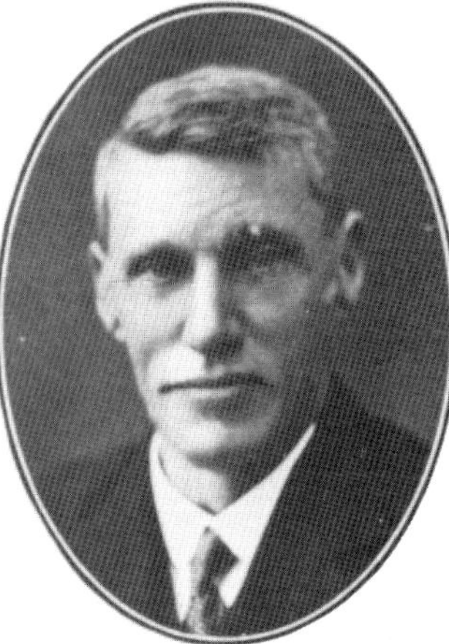

PROFESSOR J. K. JAMIESON
Fourth Dean
1918–36

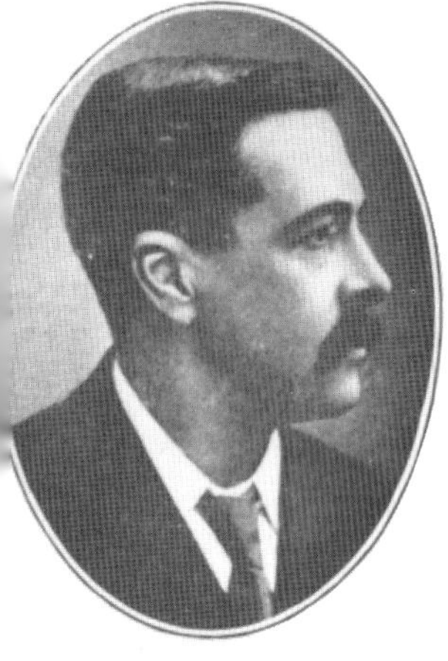

PROFESSOR A. S. GRÜNBAUM
Second Dean
1907–13

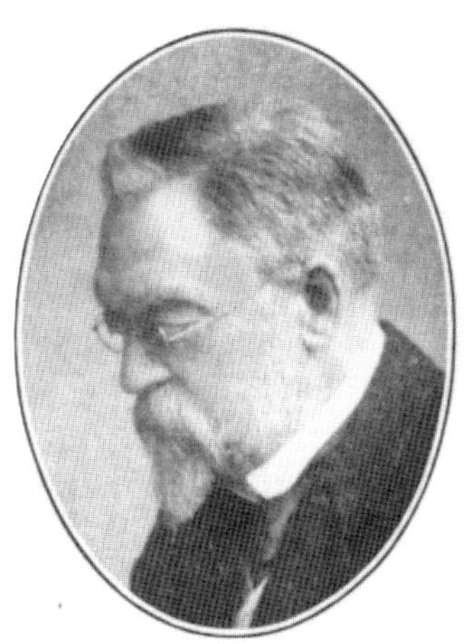

PROFESSOR J. B. HELLIER
Third Dean
1917–18

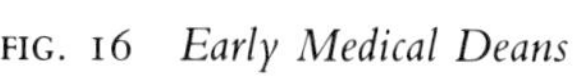

FIG. 16 *Early Medical Deans*

Dean's Office and the biology and chemistry sections were transferred to the College Library. A library catalogue was printed in 1891 and 500 library cards prepared. The 'Book of Benefactions' which had been kept by Dr Heaton was, after his death in 1880, updated by Mr Wright in 1886.

The museum of instruments benefited in 1888 by a gift from Mr Atkinson which included an old stethoscope. In 1891 Dr Braithwaite donated a pair of crotchets, a vectis and a fillet and Mr Scattergood gave two pairs of midwifery forceps, three Lisfranc's specula and three ether inhalers, two of which being those used when ether anaesthesia was introduced at the Infirmary in 1847.

It is of interest that two stills had been used illicitly in the School for many years before their use was regularised in 1890. The Inland Revenue also decided that 'the Dean should be allowed to receive for Museum and Anatomical Purposes, without bond being required, 150 gallons of methylated spirit annually'. It was obtained from Leith in thirty-gallon casks at 2/4 gallon carriage paid and was kept in a padlocked wooden erection iin the yard, the key being held by the Professor of Pathology.[36]

Overcrowding again

The number of new students entering the School in the 1880s was increasing and approaching an annual intake of fifty, which indeed it reached in 1888–89.[37] Subjects such as physiology and pathology were expanding. Such was the need for lecture space in 1889 that the Board Room of the Infirmary was used for lectures in medicine and surgery. The School was becoming uncomfortably overcrowded and there had been recurring problems with ventilation. In November 1887 a committee was set up to look into the possibility of extending the school buildings and recommended in April 1888 the purchase of land lying to the north of the School in Park Street.[38] An alternative suggestion of transferring the Department of Physiology to College Road was favoured by the committee appointed by the Council of the College, but the Board of the Medical Department resolved 'That it is not desirable permanently to separate the departments of teaching at present included in the Medical School and that it is especially undesirable to carry on the work of teaching Anatomy, and Physiology in buildings separated from one another.' It asked the Professors of Medicine, Surgery, Anatomy and Physiology and the Dean to consider various ways of altering the buildings or acquiring another site.[39]

REFERENCES

1. Asa Briggs 'The Eighteen Seventies', *The University of Leeds Review*, vol 17, no 2. 1974, pp 217–19.
2. S. T. Anning, *The General Infirmary at Leeds*, vol II, Edinburgh and London, 1966, pp 138.
3. A. N. Shimmin, *The University of Leeds, The First Half-Century*, Cambridge, 1954, pp 11–18.
4. Leeds School of Medicine Council Book 4, 19 March 1875.
5. Leeds School of Medicine Prospectuses 1864–65 to 1883–84 (in Medical Library, University of Leeds).
6. Leeds School of Medicine Council Book 4.
7. Charles Newman, *The Evolution of Medical Education in the Nineteenth Century*, London (1957).
8. Leeds School of Medicine Council Book 4, 28 April 1878.
9. Ibid, 13 May 1879.
10. Ibid, 21 May 1883.
11. Ibid, 23 August 1883 and 11 September 1883.
12. Ibid, 1 October 1883.
13. Ibid, 7 February 1884.
14. Ibid, 13 November 1883.
15. Ibid, 28 February 1884.
16. Ibid, 26 May 1884.
17. Ibid, 16 July 1884.
18. Ibid, 16 June 1882.
19. Ibid, 7 August 1884.
20. Yorkshire College Medical Department Minute Book, 6 August 1884.
21. Leeds School of Medicine, Treasurer's Book 4, 11 August 1884.
22. Yorkshire College Medical Department Minute Book, 6 November 1884 and 20 August 1885.
23. Ibid, 6 November 1884.
24. Ibid, 16 September 1884.
25. Ibid, 16 April 1885.
26. Ibid, 19 November 1885.
27. Ibid, 21 January 1886.
28. Ibid, 18 November 1886.
29. Yorkshire College Calendar, 1888–89, p 6.
30. Yorkshire College Medical Department Minute Book, 30 June 1887.
31. S. T. Anning, *The General Infirmary at Leeds*, vol II, Edinburgh and London, 1966, p 58 and Lord Moynihan, 'Days Gone By', *University of Leeds Medical Society Magazine*, vol IV, 1934, pp 88–91.
32. Yorkshire College Medical Department Minute Book, 21 July 1887.
33. Ibid, 7 June 1888.

34. Ibid, 11 December 1884.
35. Ibid, 17 February 1887.
36. Ibid, 20 June 1890.
37. Ibid, 6 June 1889.
38. Ibid, 5 April 1888.
39. Ibid, 3 May 1888.

CHAPTER SEVEN

The School in Thoresby Place

THE MOUNT PLEASANT ESTATE proved an ideal site for the proposed new School. Mount Pleasant was an attractive two-storey double-fronted house, which from Park Street, could be seen at the top of the slope between the Infirmary and St George's Church.[1] There were gardens to the sides and tenanted outbuildings at the back facing Blundell Street (Fig 17). It was owned by the Infirmary, which had acquired it together with its own site in 1862. Mr Nicholson Price, surgeon, who had retired from the School with Dr Allbutt in 1884, had been tenant for several years. A minute expressing sympathy at his death was written on 5 July 1888 and just over two months later on 18 September 1888 the Board of the Medical Department were considering the advantages of the site:

> 'The area is ample, allowing (no inconsiderable advantage) of an inner courtyard. The situation is convenient in its close proximity to the Infirmary and in its being placed at an almost equal distance between the central buildings of the College and the Railway Station. The site is a commanding one and is admirably fitted for the erection of an imposing building which would be well exposed to air and sunlight, completely detached from other erections, bounded by good streets and capable of being well drained.'

Purchase was recommended.[2] The College offered £6000, the Infirmary Board accepted, with restrictions that prevented the erection of other than College buildings, and the Draft agreement to Purchase was approved, all within the space of five weeks.[3] Payment was by instalments which were completed in July 1889.

At about this time the College wished also to build the Great Hall and Library and it was decided on 24 January 1890 to launch an appeal to the public for £40,000 'of which about £25,000 will be required for the Medical School and £15,000 for the Hall and covered way'.[4] A month later almost £25,000 had been subscribed but only a further £7000 was added by June.[5]

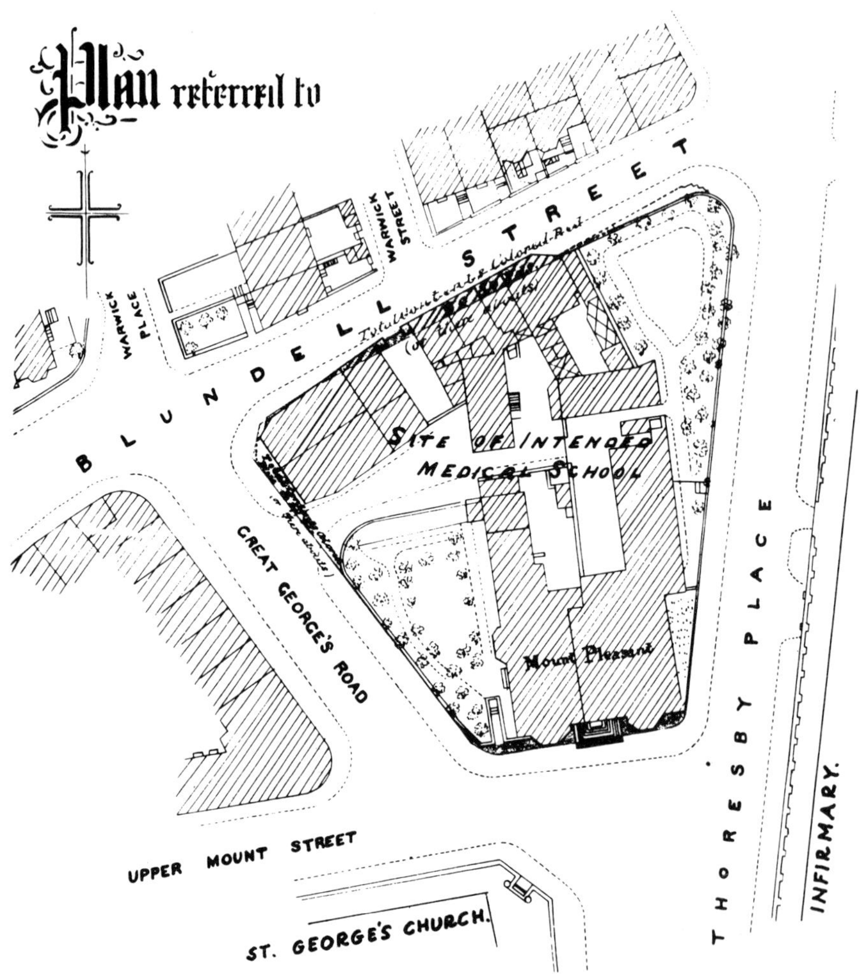

FIG. 17 *The Mount Pleasant Site*

Planning

In July Mr W. H. Thorp who had been responsible for the design of the Leeds Art Gallery, was chosen as the architect for the Medical School and later in the year he visited the schools at Newcastle, Edinburgh, Glasgow, Dublin, and Cambridge. In December 1890 he was asked for a rough estimate of the cost of a school for 400 students (assuming an annual entry of 100) with three or four lecture rooms, two to accommodate at least 220; for departments of physiology, pathology, pharmacy, anatomy, materia medica, and surgery, with museums, library, professors' and students' common rooms, dining room, lavatories, cloakrooms, and porter's living rooms.[6] On hearing that the cost without internal fittings would be £31,500 this ambitious plan was curtailed. The Board agreed that provision for an annual intake of eighty would be sufficient and that the three lecture theatres should seat 180, 100 and 80; it was also agreed to build on three sides only, leaving the fourth side (the west block) for completion at a later date.[7] The revised plans, at a cost of £25,000, were approved on 20 March 1891. The Medical School Building Committee under the chairmanship of Mr Scattergood met in the next three years with increasing frequency to deal with matters of detail and more than eighty meetings are recorded.

In the late summer of 1891 a hoarding was placed round the site, the tenants still resident on the Mount Pleasant property were given 'a week's notice to quit', the house was demolished and the materials were sold at auction by Hepper & Sons for £340; 59 square yards of spare land in Blundell Street were sold to the Corporation for road widening (see plan). The design of the building was advanced for its day. Heating was to be by low pressure steam; ventilation by a Guibal fan 6 ft in diameter, driven by a 6 hp motor, which would withdraw air from the rooms into extract ducts and propel it up the ventilation shaft of the main chimney; the windows on the south side were to have iron casements and those in the lecture theatres to have double panes; copper piping was to be used for the hot water system; the floors of the principal upper rooms to be of fireproof concrete.[8] It was at first intended to light the building by gas, with wiring installed so that future connection to an electricity supply would be possible. However, in January 1893 it was decided to install electric lighting from the beginning at a cost of about £1000 and over six hundred and fifty 16 candle-power bulbs were ordered. The question arose as to whether the School should make its own electricity or obtain

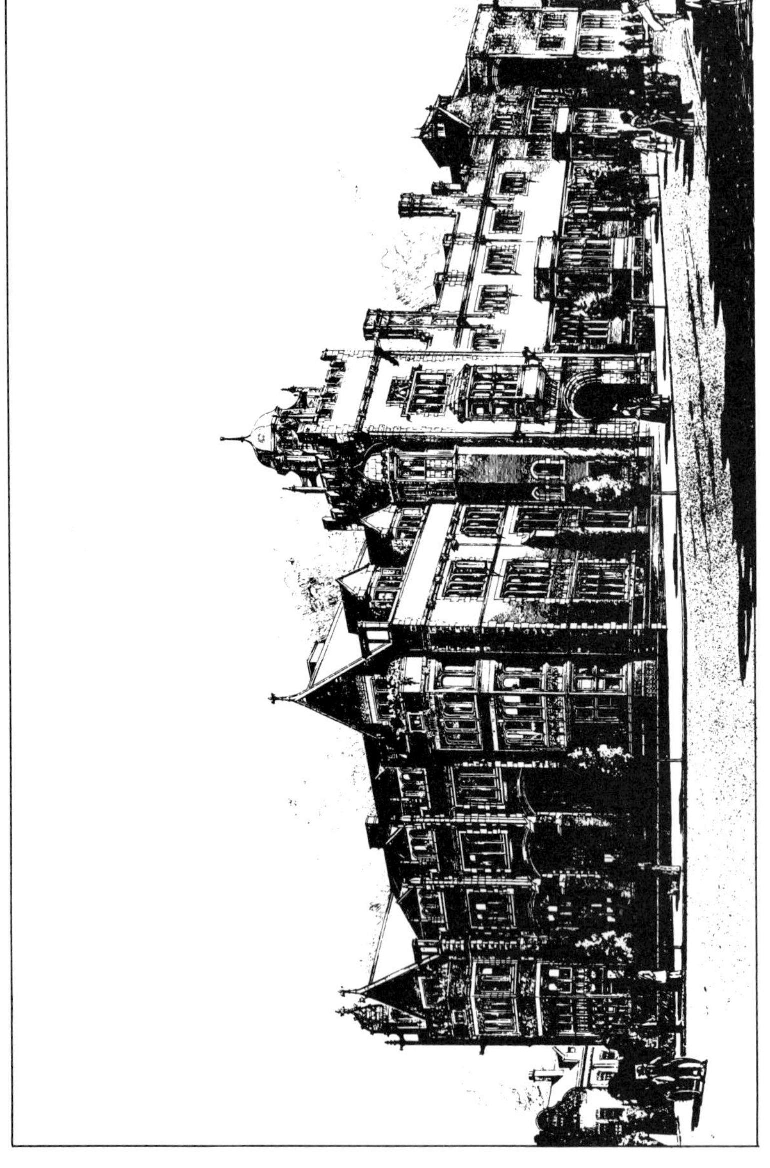

FIG. 18 *The School in Thoresby Place*

it from the House to House Electricity Company. The latter was chosen as the difference in the annual cost was estimated to be less than £5.[9] Natural roof lighting was used for dissecting room and museums.

At one stage a subway connecting the School and Infirmary was considered but the cost would have been £450 and no action was taken.[10]

Building

Tenders for the new building were invited by advertisement. In November 1891 that of W. Wilson & Sons at a contract price of £25,060 was accepted, the date of completion to be 1 July 1893 with a penalty for non-completion of £20 per week.[11] A separate tender for the heating and ventilation amounted to £1931, in the provisions of which the engine to drive the extract fan would be mounted on a wooden platform with coconut matting in order to deaden sound which might otherwise disturb the adjacent general lecture theatre.

There were certain problems with materials; the supply of Morley stone was stopped owing to a strike of quarry men — strikes occurred even in those days — and alternatives had to be found;[12] a tender for white Mansfield stone was accepted for the upper part of the Hexagon Hall.

Eighteen months had been allowed for building and in December 1892, a year having elapsed, the committee was dissatisfied with progress. They were also concerned at the irregular colour of the Burmantofts faience in the Hexagon Hall, but decided not to delay the work by removing it.[13]

During 1893 many details were settled; a telephone was to be installed in the porter's lodge with speaking tubes from there to the library and to other departments; a circular staircase was to be added to the library; air filters were to be like the specimen submitted by Mr Pridgin Teale.

In June a temporary loan of £15,000, on the security of stocks of the College, was needed for the completion of the building.[14] Furniture and fittings were considered in the autumn and in January 1894 the master key arrangements were approved and ninety-eight lockers were ordered. From February a man was employed to fire the boiler to dry out the building and the main staircase and library ceiling were strengthened. £30 was expended on forty examination desks, £40 on furniture for the

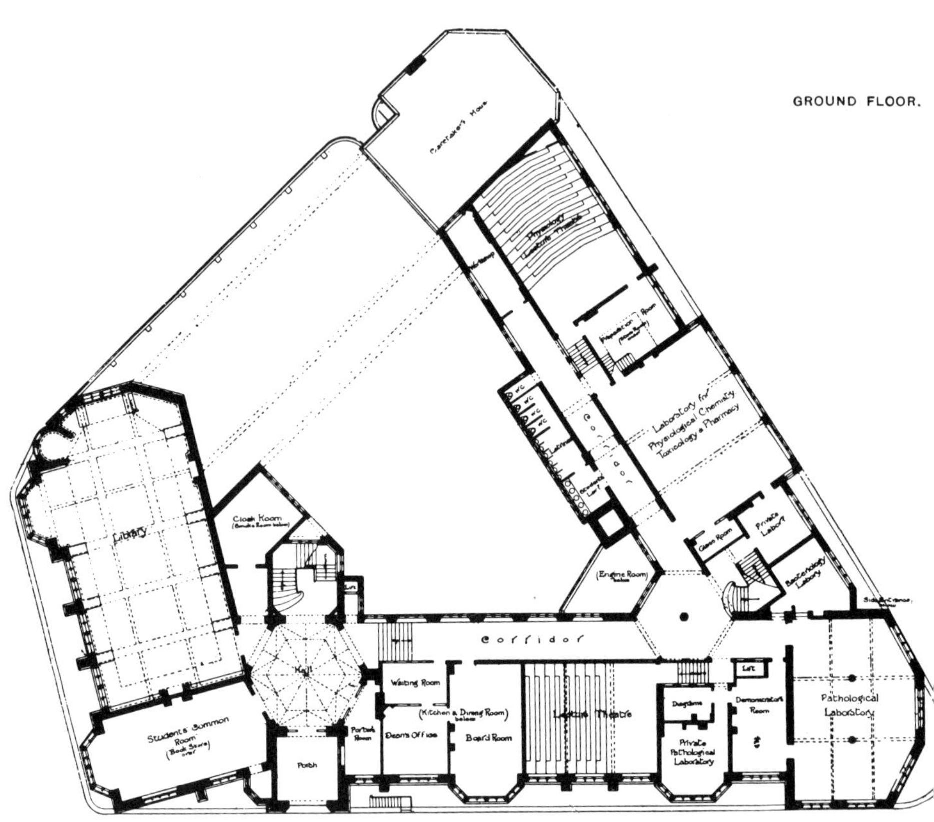

FIG. 19 *Plan of Ground Floor, Thoresby Place School*

three professors' rooms, ten tables were ordered for the dining room at £1.10.6 and forty bent wood chairs at 4/3 each.[15]

The building was sufficiently finished by the summer for Physiology to move in and the first class to be held in the new building was in histology on 28 May. Pharmacy followed quickly and the Library moved in October.

Bringing in more furniture, the fitting of blinds and a socket for the flagpole, completion of panelling, painting, decorating, and labelling of rooms in black paint continued through the summer to be ready for the opening in October. The faience work by the Burmantofts Company could not be finished in time and was deferred to the Easter vacation.

Official opening

The School was formally opened on 5 October 1894 by the Duke of York (later King George V). The Duke and Duchess had been staying at Balmoral, broke their journey in Edinburgh which they left on 4 October at 10 am to arrive in York at 2.25. There they took a special train to Garforth Station and drove to Temple Newsam where they spent the night. A careful schedule had been prepared for the day of the opening. They drove at trotting pace to the city boundary, at walking pace to the Town Hall in Victoria Square and after a ten-minute stop for a civic welcome by the Lord Mayor then proceeded by way of Cookridge Street to the Yorkshire College for a visit lasting three-quarters of an hour during which the Great Hall was opened. At 1.05 they left the College and came by Clarendon Road to Thoresby Place, to be received in the entrance porch by Principal Bodington, Mr Scattergood (the Dean) and Mr Thorp (the Architect). A gold key was presented to the Duke who then toured the building in which 1200 people were gathered: into the Hexagon Hall which he greatly admired, up the main staircase to the Pathology Museum where there was a fine collection of plants down the centre of the room and 300 visitors; thence by the side door to the Anatomy Museum and to the dissecting room filled with 400 visitors; on to the Anatomy Lecture Theatre where present students were gathered; on through the Physiology Department and back to the Library where there were 360 people in the area and in the gallery a further 100 and a band which had been playing music. The opening ceremony is said to have taken half a minute. Lord Ripon invited the

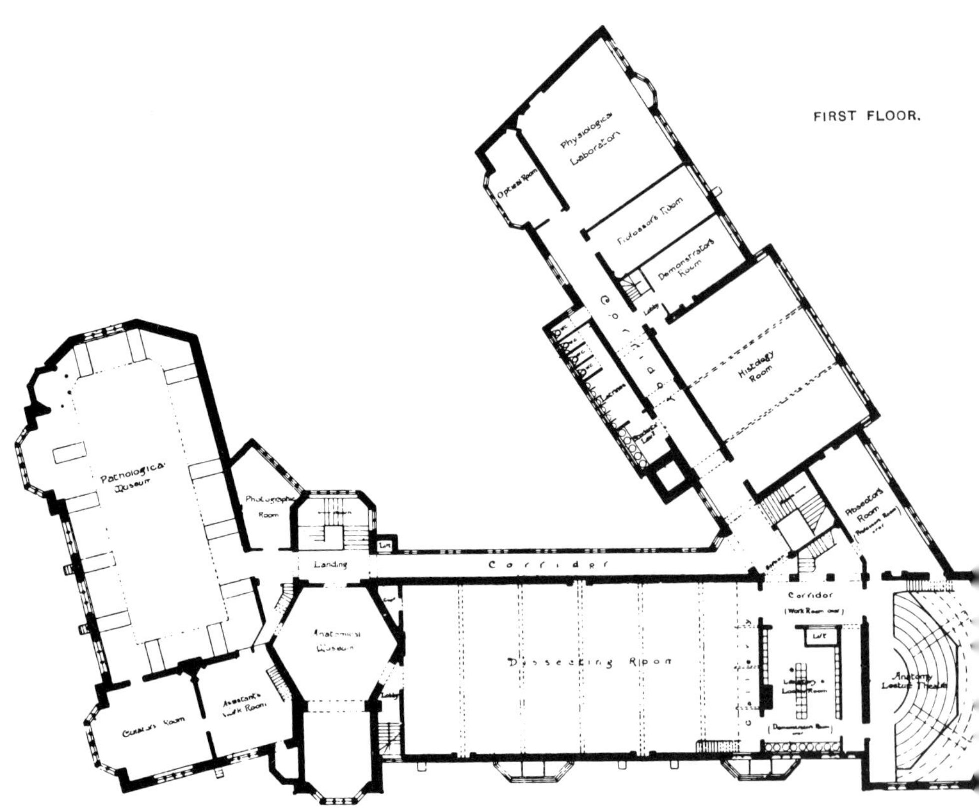

FIG. 20 *Plan of First Floor, Thoresby Place School*

Duke to speak and the Duke said 'I have great pleasure in declaring the new Medical School of the Yorkshire College open and I wish it every prosperity'. The visit to the School had taken 35 minutes and after a late lunch at the Town Hall the Duke and Duchess left Leeds at 3.30.[16]

It had been something of a civic occasion. When they arrived they had passed under an arch constructed of bread loaves in Commercial Street, a photograph of which is to be found in Dr Anning's book *The General Infirmary at Leeds.*[17] It had been intended to give the bread afterwards to the poor but it rained. It was presumably fine in the evening for bright scenes in the streets were described.

On Monday 8 October in the afternoon the School was open to the public and in the evening a Conversazione was held to which were invited the Lord Mayor, the staff of the College, medical men in Yorkshire and all past students of the School. Demonstrations, experiments and entertainment were provided. It is unfortunate that the cylinder bearing a recorded message made by the Dean into the receiver of a gramophone has been lost. Refreshments during the evening included 'tea and coffee, bread and butter, sandwiches, biscuits, lemonade, ices and cup'. The Royal Reception Committee which had had sixteen meetings finally arranged a 'Workman's Supper' at 2/- per head for the 300 men who could be certified by their employers as having worked on College buildings for at least a year.[18]

Although the building was almost a year late — delays occurred in those days also — it was worth waiting for, and is now listed as of architectural or historical interest. The architect's drawing (Fig 18) shows the south and east elevations. These aspects of the exterior are the most attractive. It is built of stone and red brick. Stone carvings of animal heads and gargoyles, partially obscured by the grime of Leeds and eroded in places, are no doubt less obvious than when the building was new, but together with shields and floral designs can still be seen by the observant eye. The main entrance is on the east side at the foot of the tower and above it is an attractive oriel window. At a higher level on the tower the arms of the Yorkshire College, with the motto 'Et Augebitur Scientia', are carved in stone. The tower has an embattled parapet and above it a wooden lantern and finial. The Library and Student Common Rooms (later taken into the library) occupy the ground floor on the south side. Two minor turrets may be seen, one octagonal with perpendicular panelled sides and lead ogee dome at the west corner of the library and a

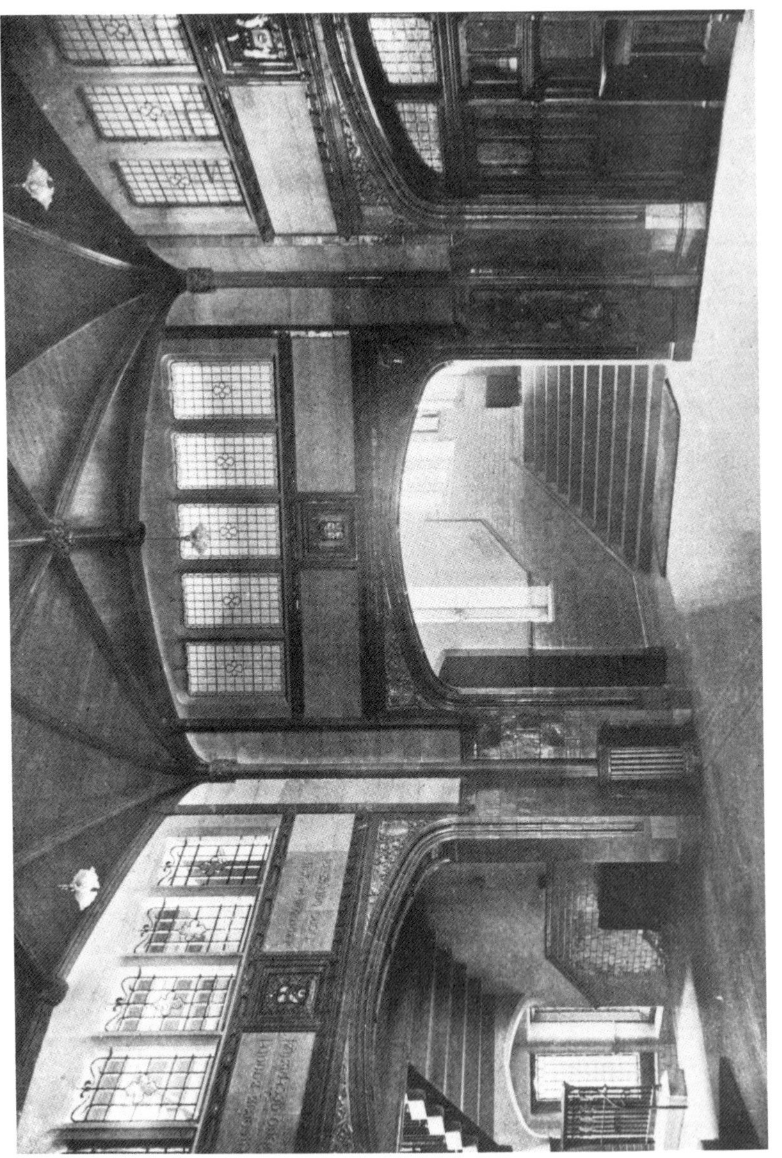

FIG. 21 *The Hexagon Hall*

smaller one close against the south side of the tower. To the right of the entrance the first of the bay windows belongs to the Board Room.

The plans of the principal floors (Figs 19 and 20) show the general layout of the rooms. The Hexagon Hall (Fig 21) is entered through an open archway. It is unique in design and repays close inspection. The arcaded sides of the hall are covered in glazed Burmantofts tiling greenish in colour. The upper part of the walls are in white stone with clerestory windows admitting 'borrowed light'; the roof is oak, vaulted and ribbed; the floor is marble mosaic. Above the five arches are to be seen the coats of arms of the Victoria University, the Royal College of Physicians, the Yorkshire College, the Royal College of Surgeons and the City of Leeds. Above the centre archway leading to the principal staircase (Fig 22) is the inscription 'AEGROTOS SANATE, LEPROSOS PURGATE: DONO ACCEPISTIS, DONO DATE'. It was chosen by Mr Scattergood and is a quotation from Theodore Beza's Latin translation of Matthew 10:8, which may be rendered 'Heal the sick, cleanse the lepers; freely you have received, freely give'. Professor W. G. Arnott has drawn attention to the omission of the middle two exhortations (mortuos suscitate, daemonia ejicite) to raise the dead and cast out devils, 'two occupations less relevant to a Medical School'. Seen with the inscription in Fig 22 are: the shield of the Yorkshire College, adopted by the School of Medicine as its own; the clerestory windows; and part of the Burmantofts faience with vine leaves and grapes above the left of the arch and oak leaves and acorns above the right. From the top of the short flight of steps which lead from the Hexagon Hall to the Board Room, it was customary for many years for the Dean to read examination results to students crowded into the hall below. From the Board Room the corridor leads on to the Small Hexagon Hall (Fig 23) which has a central pillar and radiating arches.

The Library (Fig 24) is entered from the Hexagon Hall and is a fine room. It is partially subdivided into alcoves by the oak bookcases, has good proportions (72 ft long, 35 ft wide and 18 ft high) having a balcony and wrought-iron balustrade at 10 ft. The beams supporting the ceiling are encased in oak and between them the plaster is moulded in a geometrical pattern.[19] It is indeed one of the finest rooms in the University and has been used for lectures, degree ceremonies, receptions, and for Medical Balls in the nineteen thirties and again in 1978.

The original Pathology Museum (Fig 25) situated above the Library is also a room of some character. The Anatomy Theatre (Fig 26) is

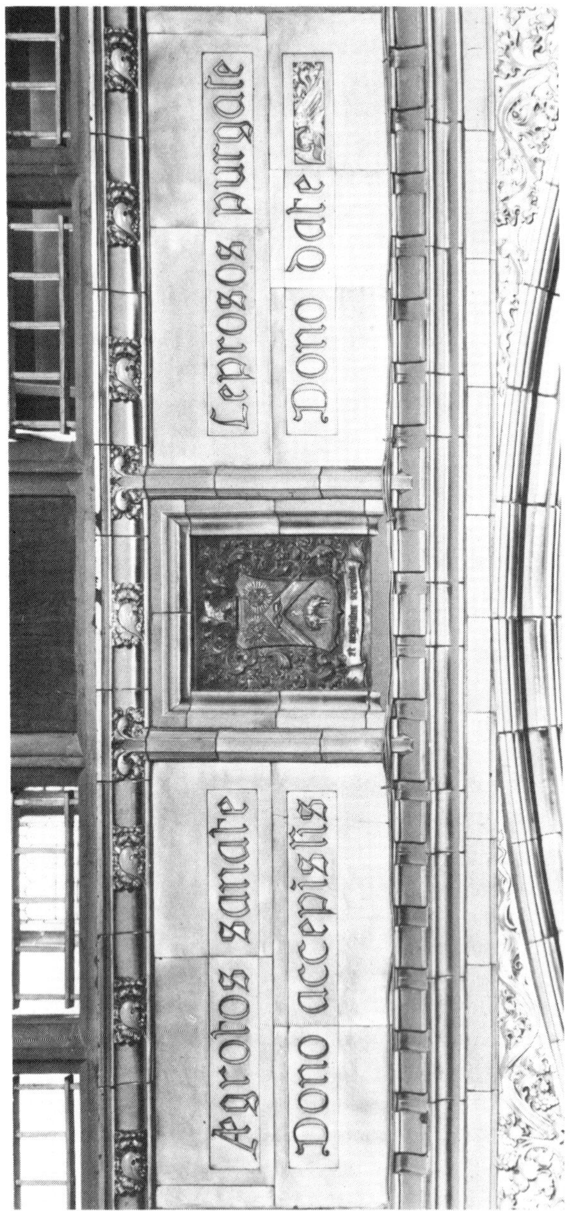

FIG. 22 *The Shield and Motto, Clerestory Windows and part of the Burmantofts Faience*

remarkable for its steep rake; originally the seating was none too comfortable especially for those with long legs, and the book rest was so narrow and sloping that going to sleep during a lecture could be disastrous.

These various illustrations will evoke memories for generations of graduates who received part of their training in this building and many who have worked in more modern buildings may echo the view of the *Leeds Mercury* at the opening: 'There is a compactness about the premises that gives it an air of comfort.'

Many stories could be told of the Refectory in the basement. For over eighty years from its opening in February 1895 it proved as was intended 'a great convenience and saver of time', but also a meeting place where students, over cups of tea and coffee, talked of work and other things (its only rival in this respect being the dissecting room). At the outset Mrs Bennett was in charge, catering and managing at 10/- per week aided by a young girl at 3/- per week and a waitress at 6/-; the latter, the committee insisted, must be a married woman. They would have preferred a waiter, but Mrs Bennett said 'that would be more expensive and there would be so much less work done'. Beer was served but Mrs Bennett had private instructions to serve only gentlemen taking lunch and not more than half a pint to anyone.[20]

After the first six months the accounts were almost in balance but most often thereafter they were in deficit. It was discovered in 1897, as has been found since, that increasing the prices or making a table charge produces consumer resistance. Then the price of beer was raised from 1½d to 2d per glass and wages amounted to only 20 per cent or so of income instead of the 40 per cent or 50 per cent or much higher figure of recent years.[21]

White tablecloths and waitress service disappeared with the Second World War. In the war years the manageress, who slept on the premises, used to store the chocolate and sweet rations in her room, to be dispensed only to her favourites; some people felt it encouraged the mice. A disastrous period followed when outside caterers were given the franchise, but they had not reckoned on the uneven trading and the food went from bad to worse. There was relief and considerable improvement when the University Catering Officer took over. In the nineteen sixties and seventies the Refectory, always an intimate place, took on a new cheerfulness displaying pictures lent by the Department of Fine Art and it

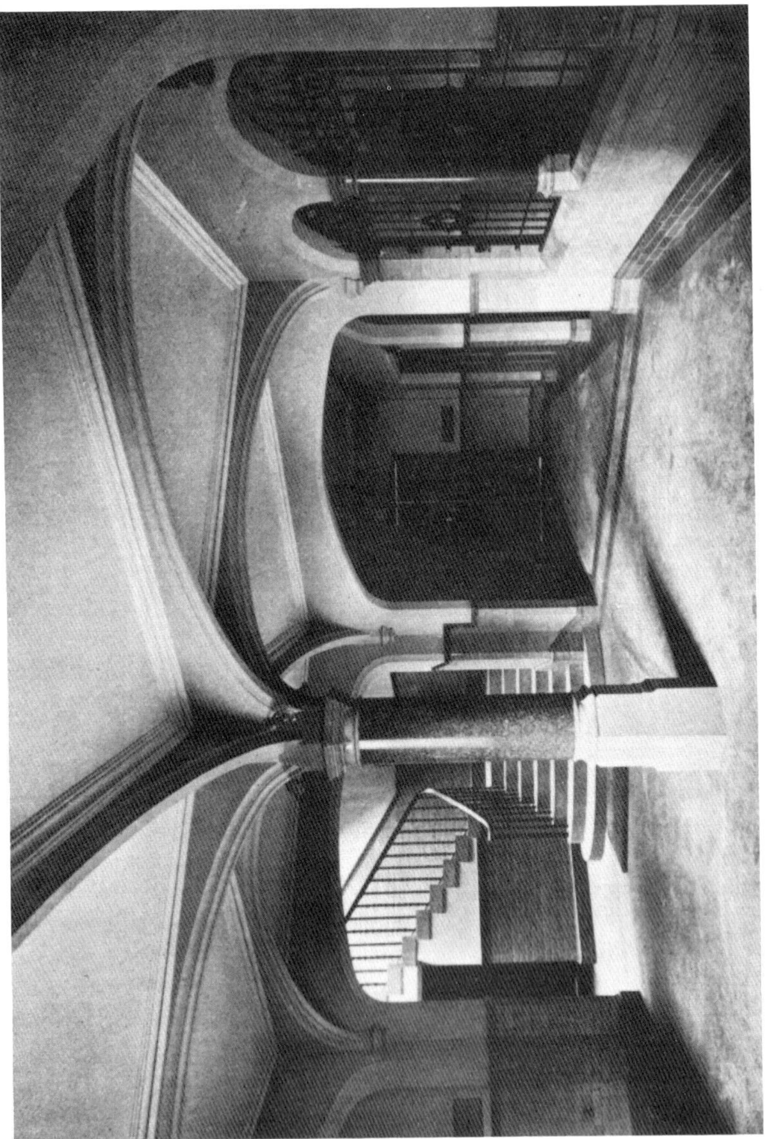

FIG. 23 *The Small Hexagon Hall*

continued to serve students and staff until the building was largely vacated in 1977.

The new school was not without its troubles. The number of student entries had decreased somewhat from the high point in 1888 and consequently the revenue to the College was less. It was reported in 1896 that the Medical Department finances were in deficit for the second year in succession; College finances were also strained and it was agreed that the one-third of gross fees set aside for the part-time professors and lecturers be not taken until fixed salaries and running expenses had been met. In effect they agreed to accept and divide what was left over. The Dean was quick to point out however that lest this should be construed as profit sharing, which was against the constitution of the College, 'no profit can fairly be said to be made until the staff like other servants of the College shall have been properly remunerated for their services'. At the same time it was recommended that 'as the Professor of Physiology devotes his whole time to the College his stipend should be raised from £300 to £350'. However, staff in other parts of the College receiving over £400 per year made offers of diminution, Principal Bodington by £100 and Professor Smithells by £150.[22]

Economies started early — some of the 16 candle-power bulbs were changed to 8 candle-power in October 1894, and when in 1898 the House to House Electricity Supply Company gave notice that it would change from 100 volt to 200 volt supply the House Committee asked 'what compensation if any they proposed to make for throwing out of use our present lamps'.[23] Some noise from the dissecting room above and heat from the boiler house below were reported in the general lecture theatre. Remedies were needed for the smoke that found its way into the dissecting room and valves were introduced into the duct-work to prevent odours from the anatomy cellars reaching the Physiology Department.

In February 1900 Mr Thomas Scattergood died. He had been associated with the School for over fifty-four years (see Chapter 11); it was decided that his portrait should be hung in the Board Room (it is now on Level 7 in the Worsley Building) and the Scattergood Prize in Obstetrics was instituted. Professor de Burgh Birch (Fig 16) became Dean.[24]

Bacteriology, as a separate course, had started in the summer of 1894, consisting of twelve lessons each of three hours of laboratory teaching. The fee was £4.4.0, the student to find his own microscope.[25] One room

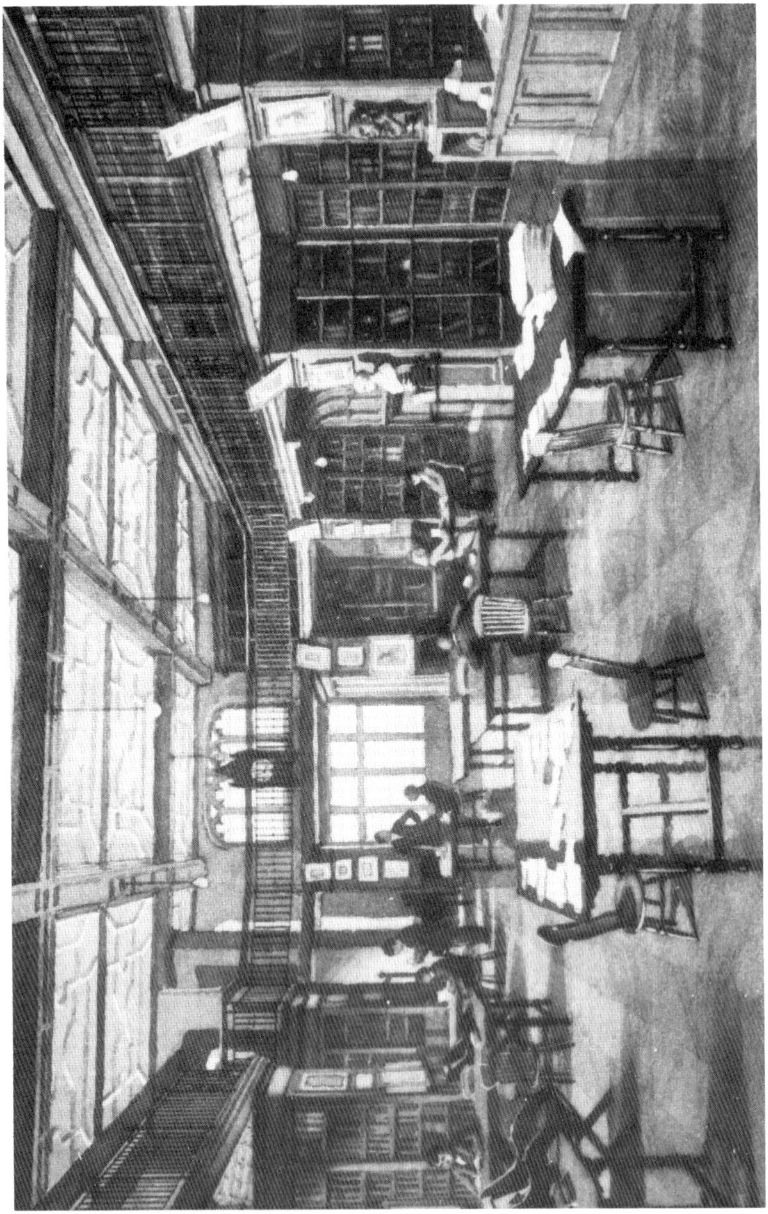

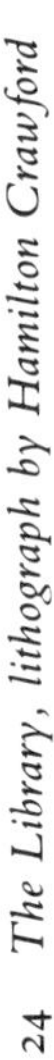

FIG. 24 *The Library, lithograph by Hamilton Crawford*

is shown on the Plan (Fig 19) as devoted to Bacteriology. The subject was expanding rapidly however and in 1902 it was even suggested that the Board Room be used. In the same year the Report Book states that the Professors of Anatomy and of Pathology were 'willing to resign in favour of whole time professors when funds are available', but in 1902–03 students were fewer, only thirty-four composition tickets being sold compared with fifty-one the previous year. In 1905 a new building for Pathology was suggested on the fourth side of the courtyard. Eventually additional accommodation for Pathology and Bacteriology was found in St George's House on the other side of St George's Road.

The University

The University received its Charter on 25 April 1904 and an Act to merge the Yorkshire College in the University of Leeds and to transfer all property, etc, received Royal Assent on 24 June 1904. In preparation for the 1904–05 Session a committee was set up on 26 February 1904 to consider degree examinations in the University of Leeds. On the establishment of the University the Medical Department of the Yorkshire College became known as the Faculty of Medicine of the University. A smooth transition was effected. Professor Birch remained Dean and as such received £50 per annum. In 1905 the Dean requested the services of a shorthand typist for a half day per week, while in 1912 a Sub-Librarian and Clerk was appointed to combine oversight of the Library and the official correspondence of the Dean and Academic Sub-Dean at £2 per week, also a boy to assist at 5/-.[26] Student numbers were reported to be increasing again in 1906.

Staff

The most flamboyant surgical figure of the eighteen nineties was probably Arthur W. Mayo-Robson. As a student he was an avid collector of prizes and later of awards and decorations and used his opportunities to the full. He was one of the pioneers of surgery of the upper abdomen especially of the biliary tract, but was perhaps at his best in operating on the acute abdomen, using quickness and skill combined with a knowledge of when to stop. According to J. F. Dobson 'his

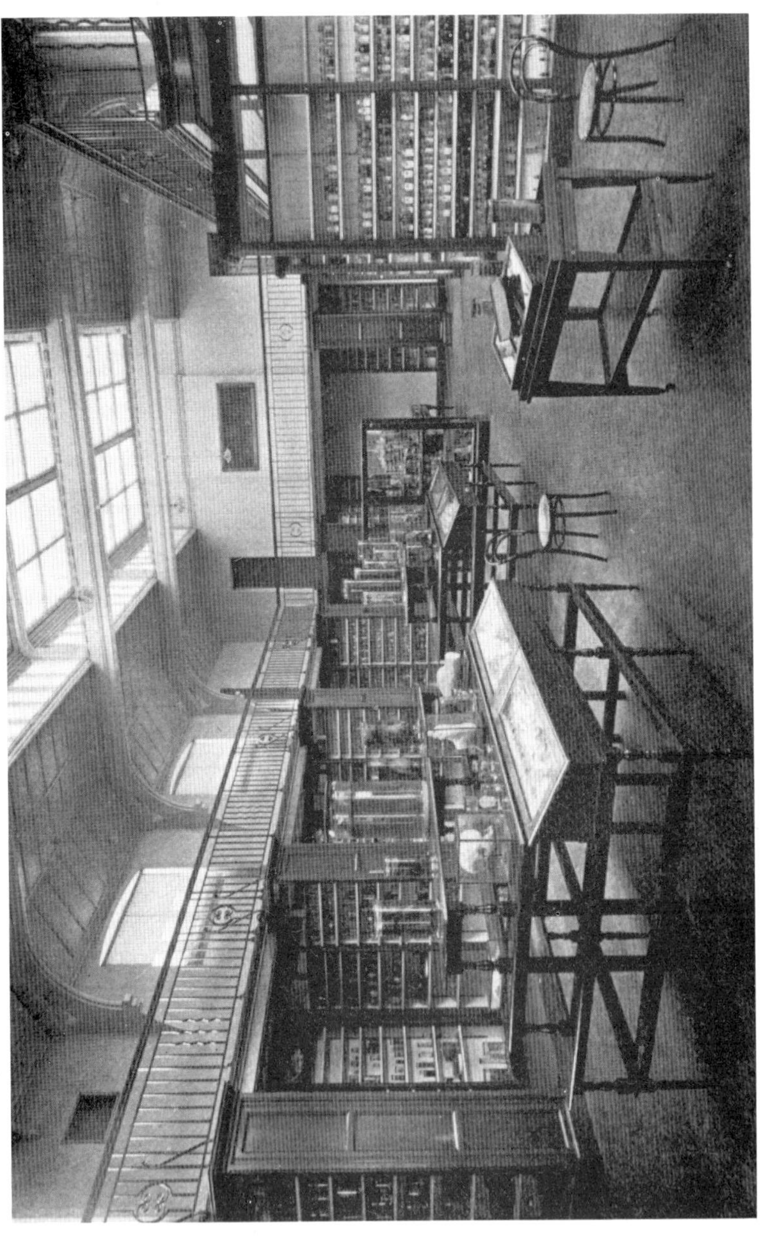

FIG. 25 *The Pathology Museum (later Histology Class Room, now a Microbiology Laboratory)*

orthopaedic work (when he condescended to practise orthopaedics) was good' and he was operating successfully on torn cartilages of the knee before his contemporaries.[27] He was Professor of Surgery from 1890 to 1899 but his move to London in 1902 proved a disappointment. He received an honorary DSc (Leeds) in 1904, was knighted in 1908 and gave useful service in the 1914–18 war.

The names of two professors of surgery in the decade 1900–10 are commemorated in prizes: Edward Ward (Fig 15) in the prize in surgical anatomy awarded in the final year and Harry Littlewood (Fig 15) 1904–10 in the prize in anatomy awarded in the second year. Littlewood had a thumb missing but was a good operator and pioneered the fore-quarter amputation. The instructional block in the Infirmary was furnished in his memory, the hall being known as the Littlewood Hall.

Undoubtedly the Leeds graduate who attained the highest honours and worldwide acclaim was Berkeley George Andrew Moynihan. A student of the School from 1883 he took the London MB degree and MRCS in 1887, was dresser to McGill and house surgeon to Mayo-Robson. He was Lecturer in Surgery from 1890 to 1909, Professor of Clinical Surgery from 1910 to 1925 and Professor of Surgery from 1925 to 1927. He was President of the Royal College of Surgeons of England for six years from 1926 to 1931. His main contribution was in the perfection of techniques of abdominal surgery in the surgery of the spleen, gall-bladder, stomach, duodenum, and intestines. He reached the pinnacle of success by hard work; he was an orator but perfected his speeches before giving them. He became KB (1912), CB (1917), KCMG (1918), Baronet (1922), Baron (1929).

His nephew Andrew Moynihan Claye, Professor of Obstetrics 1936–61 became another provincial president of a Royal College, in this case PRCOG. He was a cultured man, quoted poetry, and sang in the Leeds Festival Chorus and was one of the few of his time who gave some teaching in contraception.

Leeds has had its good physicians too, but though practice has been sound, progress, apart from Allbutt, has been less spectacular. In the specialties, J. P. Bibby in venereology and J. T. Ingram in dermatology were primarily excellent physicians.

Leeds has continued to attract and to produce surgeons of calibre from Braithwaite and Flint to Goligher and others. Many, especially of the earlier surgeons, had surgical instruments made to their own design and in the main it would be true that these have been gentler to the tissues and neater than those in use elsewhere at the time.

For those who were students in the period 1936–64 when Archibald Durward was Professor of Anatomy, his name will evoke many memories: of lectures delivered in inimitable style with perfect control and use of language, lectures which 'pointed the moral and adorned the tale'; of a curriculum carefully worked out which then invariably ran smoothly; of stimulation usually kindly, sometimes scathing. He was very much a University man and was Pro-Vice-Chancellor in 1959–61. The Durward Travelling Scholarship was endowed by subscription and his books form the nucleus of the departmental library which bears his name.

Students

In February 1894 the principle of making one half day per term a College holiday was approved, but by March the approval was for two half days per term for inter-collegiate matches.[28]

In March also the Board noted the proposed formation of a Students' Council. By June it had been born and was granted the use of the Dean's Room for meetings, management of the Common Room and Smoking Room in the new school and was allowed to 'levy a subscription not exceeding 1/- per year to pay for newspapers'; it had a representative on the Refectory Committee.[29] It took its duties seriously and in July wrote to the Librarian complaining of members of staff 'having out a large number of text books and retaining them an unduly long time'.[30]

In 1897 a fives court was built in the quadrangle with money raised by students and the Board arranged for a dry urinal 'in the angle of the yard near the fives court'.[31] The SRC has looked after students' interests ever since.

The Medical Society has had variable fortunes over the years with occasional gaps in continuity but has often provided substantial programmes of lectures, debates, film shows, and social functions. The first Annual Dinner of Leeds Medical Students was held in the Victoria Hotel in 1880 with an attendance of between twenty and thirty. Attendance grew to 110 in 1886, when Sir Spencer Wells, an old student of the school, was in the chair.[32] The dinners were distinct from the Inaugural Dinners held at the beginning of the session — and mentioned in the last

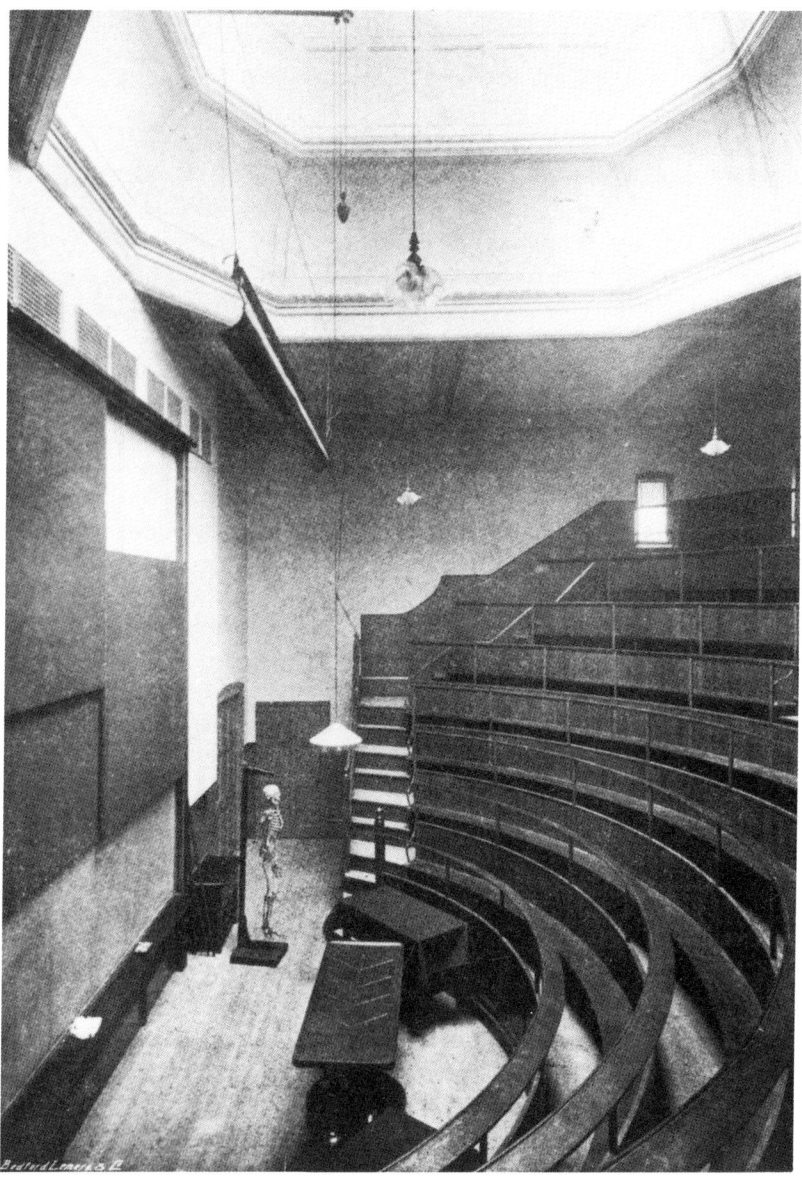

FIG. 26 *The Anatomy Theatre, 1897*

chapter. The tradition of dinners for past and present students has continued through the Thoresby Place period.

Women students

Dr Anning has drawn attention in a previous publication to the struggle of women to gain admission to medicine.[33] The first recorded application was from a Miss Colbourne in 1865. The minutes of 14 October state 'Resolved that the application of Miss Colbourne to attend lectures at this School be refused'.

The Board of the Medical Department on 2 June 1893 discussed informally whether there should be some provision of accommodation for women students in the new building and 'members present expressed themselves favourably of it being brought before the Building Committee' but a week later the question was postponed *sine die* as it was reported there was no provision for the separate teaching of women at the Infirmary. In 1895 application was made by Mrs Gilmore-Cox to attend lectures on medicine and surgery but in June this was refused as 'on enquiry she had not passed any examinations required for a diploma'.[34]

In 1897 Miss Laura Veale of Harrogate applied for admission to the School and the Dean replied stating 'there are no arrangements which enable women students to take anatomy at the Medical School'. Miss Veale then pointed out 'It seems only reasonable that I, who have been a student of the college for the past 2 sessions should have the same facilities for continuing the medical course as the men who have been my fellow students for that time'. The Board of the Medical Department on 24 September 1897, however resolved 'that the Medical Board regret that the arrangements for the Medical School render it impossible to admit Miss Veale to the classes she wishes to attend'.[35] Miss Veale qualified at the Royal Free Hospital and in 1904 became the first woman resident at the Hospital for Women and Children in Leeds.

On 26 May 1899 it was noted that there was one woman in the bacteriology class. A few others were admitted during the next ten years to study individual subjects in the school but not to the Infirmary until in 1910, following repeated pressure from the Faculty over the course of four years the Board of Governors at last agreed.

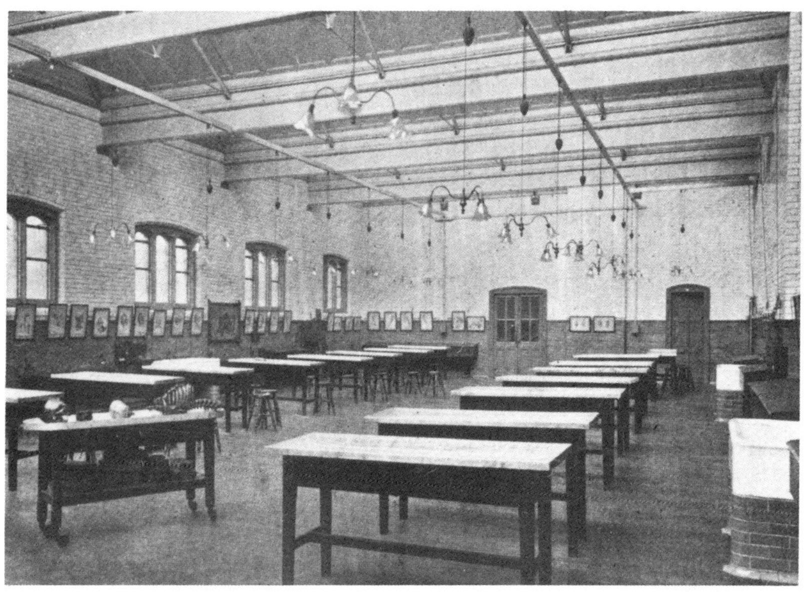

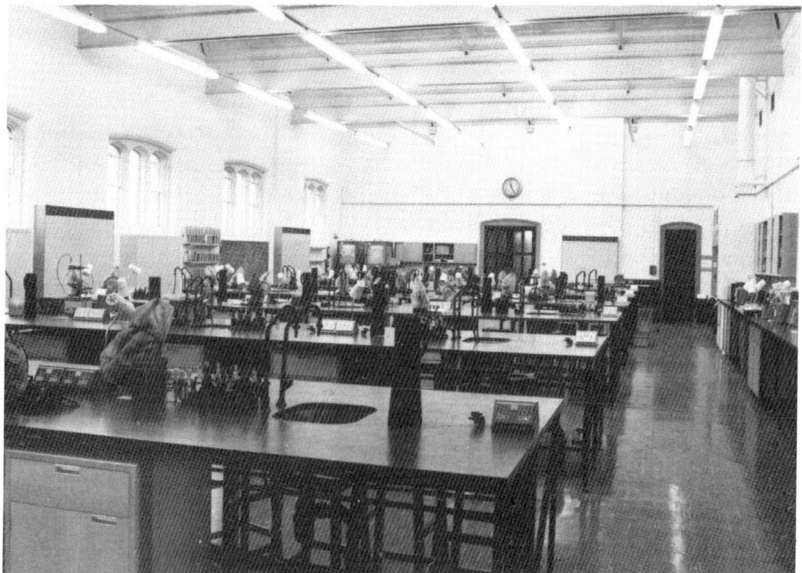

FIG. 27 *Dissecting Room in 1897; the same room as a Microbiology Laboratory, 1981*

Dr Anning reports: 'A problem arose in 1914 in connection with the dresser on duty in the Infirmary Casualty Room who went out with the ambulance. Should the "Lady Dresser" who was about to come on duty do this work? It was decided that it was not advisable for her to do so. A motor ambulance had just been presented to the Infirmary which made the duty less unsuitable for a woman student as previously there had been complaints from casualty dressers that when out with the ambulance their only responsibility had been to hold the horse's head.

'By March 1914 women students were allowed in the whole of the surgical out-patient department and in 1916 Miss Dorothy Priestley became the first woman house surgeon at the Infirmary.' The proportion of women students increased considerably during the 1914–18 war. Professor Jamieson in 1918 requested the appointment of a temporary part-time demonstrator (woman) 'as there are about 40–50 students in the Anatomy Department and about half are women'.[36]

By this time a separate women's common room had been provided; it was above the men's common room with an entrance from the mezzanine floor of the main staircase through a short stretch of the library gallery and up two steps. The doors were noisy and the floor of the gallery creaked thus providing a distraction to male readers in the library below who would momentarily glance upwards to see which lady was entering or leaving the common room. The room itself was attractive, carpeted, received the sun from early morning to mid-afternoon and looked across Thoresby Place to the Infirmary and down to the old School and the fire station in Park Street.

When in 1956 the need for more space for the library became urgent the adjacent common rooms were the obvious target and would provide it most conveniently: so the women's common room became the basic science section of the library. The men's and women's common rooms were rebuilt at that time over a refectory extension which encroached on the courtyard. The new women's common room was entered from the upper 'hanging' corridor and was long and narrow and a poor exchange for their former room. In 1968 the common rooms moved yet again to the prefabricated Lipman Building which provided jointly for both men and women.

The proportion of women had varied over the years again reaching almost half in the mid-nineteen seventies.

The Centenary — 1931

Celebrations were held for two days.[37] Delegates were invited from other universities, seventeen of which were represented; also from the Royal Colleges of Surgeons in England, Edinburgh and Ireland and the Royal Faculty of Glasgow; from London Medical Schools, the medical branches of the Armed Forces, the Society of Apothecaries, the Lister Institute, the MRC, the Royal Society, and the BMA. On Tuesday evening 30 June 1931 there were two functions running in parallel: an Old Students' Dinner at the Queen's Hotel and a Civic Reception in the Art Gallery.

On Wednesday 1 July an Honorary Degree Ceremony was held in the Great Hall at 11 am. Eight honorary degrees were awarded; included amongst the recipients were Dr Arthur Hawkyard (Lord Mayor), Emeritus Professor A. G. Barrs, Lord Dawson of Penn, Sir John Bland Sutton, and Sir Fred Gowland Hopkins, PRS. The *Yorkshire Post* reported 'The blaze of doctoral scarlet was dominant everywhere, but mingled with it were green and gold, sober black and rich wine colour, the Royal blue and silver of scores of academic robes'.[38] As the Duke of Devonshire remarked it was a scene in vivid contrast to the 'casual and unobtrusive beginning'. A luncheon for invited guests was arranged by the Leeds and West Riding Medico-Chirurgical Society at the Great Northern Hotel.

At 3 pm the Chancellor and the Dean received guests in the Library of the Medical School and demonstrations were on view in various departments, while in the Infirmary six wards, the operating theatres, kitchens, and laundry were on view. There were demonstrations also in the Dental School. Tea was available in the Anatomy Department and in the Nurses' Dining Room.

In the evening there was a University Dinner in the Queen's Hotel and this was followed by a University Ball in the Great Hall from 9 pm to 2 am. The band played from the gallery and the stage was used for sitting out. At the foot of the stage were a large number of plants with coloured electric bulbs amongst them. Academic dress was worn for the Ball and a light supper was available in the Physics Department. This consisted of sandwiches, savouries, eg lobster patties and sardines on toast, sweets, ices, and drinks: tea and coffee, claret cup, cider cup, and still lemonade.

A Centenary booklet of fifty-four pages was produced, which contained a fifteen-page short history of the School compiled at short notice by Dr Frank Hellier from his father's notes.

Those in the School in the nineteen-thirties will remember Mr Taylor, the Secretary, who under great secrecy allowed students to see their examination marks: no great harm appeared to be done; his successor was Mr Aitken. They will remember too the cheerful nod and 'Good morning, Doctor' from Mr Leonard Braithwaite to every medical student he met in the Infirmary corridor; will remember the speed of Mr Flint's operating, with two patients in the theatre and one in the anaesthetic room, all at the same time.

Others present in the war years may look back on fire watching on the roof at night, and recall how Paddy, the porter, was dismissed for drinking the alcohol from laboratory shelves. Arthur Wood succeeded him.

REFERENCES

1. S. T. Anning, *The General Infirmary at Leeds*, vol 1, Edinburgh and London, 1963, Fig 37.
2. Yorkshire College, Board of the Medical Department, Minutes, 18 September 1888.
3. Yorkshire College, Committee on the Medical Department, Committee Book 3, 24 October 1888.
4. Yorkshire College, Committee on Building Plans, Committee Book 4, 24 January 1890.
5. Yorkshire College, Canvassing Committee, Committee Book 4, 24 February 1890 and 10 June 1890.
6. Yorkshire College, Medical School Plans Committee, Committee Book 4, 22 December 1890.
7. Ibid, 23 January 1891, and 6 February 1891.
8. *The Builder*, 8 July 1893, p 30.
9. Yorkshire College, Medical Building Committee, Committee Book 5, 6 February 1893.
10. Ibid, Committee Book 4, 10 May 1892.
11. Ibid, 24 November 1891.
12. Ibid, 21 July 1892.
13. Ibid, Committee Book 5, 20 January 1893.
14. Yorkshire College, Board of the Medical Department, Minutes, 30 June 1893.
15. Yorkshire College, Medical Building Committee, Committee Book 5, 11 May 1894 and 29 June 1894.
16. *Leeds Mercury*, 6 October 1894.
17. S. T. Anning, *The General Infirmary at Leeds*, vol 1, Edinburgh and London, 1963, Fig 38.
18. W. K. J. Walls, 'The Leeds Medical School in Thoresby Place', *University of Leeds Review*, vol 20, 1977, pp 192–212.
19. Anonymous, 'The Leeds School of Medicine, being the Medical Department of the Yorkshire College, Victoria University' (undated — *c* 1897).
20. Leeds Medical School, Miscellaneous Committee Minutes, Refectory Committee, 11 and 16 February 1895.

21. Ibid, 8 October 1897.
22. Yorkshire College, Medical School House Committee Minutes, 16 March 1896.
23. Ibid, 25 June 1898.
24. Ibid, 6 July 1900.
25. Yorkshire College, Board of Medical Department, Minutes, 13 June 1894.
26. University of Leeds Archives, Miscellaneous Papers.
27. Obituary: Arthur Mayo-Robson, *University of Leeds Medical Society Magazine*, vol 4, 1934, pp 4–6.
28. Yorkshire College, Board of Medical Department, Minutes, 23 February and 30 March 1894.
29. Ibid, 29 June 1894.
30. Ibid, 26 July 1894.
31. Yorkshire College, Medical School House Committee Minutes, 9 July 1897.
32. Leeds School of Medicine, The Annual Dinner Minute Book 1880–92.
33. S. T. Anning, *The History of Medicine in Leeds*, Leeds 1980, pp 151–2.
34. Yorkshire College Medical Department Minute Book, 28 June 1895.
35. Ibid, 24 September 1897.
36. University of Leeds Archives, Miscellaneous Papers.
37. University of Leeds Archives, School of Medicine, Centenary Chest.
38. *Yorkshire Post*, 2 July 1931.

CHAPTER EIGHT

Clinical Instruction and Medical Qualifications

THE INCORPORATION of the Medical School into the Yorkshire College in 1884 gave rise to some discussion about the fees paid by students for clinical teaching in the Infirmary. The fees for pre-clinical teaching were, of course, now paid to the College which paid the lecturers. The Faculty of the Infirmary recommended in August 1884 that a composition fee of forty guineas for clinical teaching for three years should be paid, on entrance, to the Treasurer of the Infirmary and divided between the physicians and the surgeons. The courses, medical and surgical, could be paid for individually but this was much more expensive. On this basis the fees charged for surgical teaching were greater than for medical and the physicians strongly disapproved. Dr Allbutt, shortly before his retirement, wrote a long letter to the Board of the Infirmary expressing his views. He did not think it wise for the Board to receive the fees and so take on responsibility for the teaching which would be better borne by the Yorkshire College. He did not think it right that the fees for surgical courses should be higher than those for the medical and wrote: '. . . that a thriving and considerable school of medicine is to flourish and increase, not in the strength of one department or another, but in the full development of all'. This letter achieved nothing.

It was not until June 1910 that the clinical teaching at the Infirmary was transferred to the control of the University and each member of staff engaged in teaching became a member of the Board of the Faculty of Medicine of the University with an annual stipend from that body to which the fees were now paid. This seems to have resulted from information from the Dean on 1 March 1910 'that there was a reasonable probability that a grant might be obtained for the School from the Board of Education provided that the clinical work at the Infirmary could be brought within the scope of their regulations for the clinical institution. As a sum of £800 to £1000 was involved it was highly desirable that some arrangement for so large an addition to the resources of the School should be effected, whether by enlarging the membership of the Board so as to include thereon members of the Infirmary staff at present not members of the Board as well, or in some other way.' On 7 June 1910 there was: 'Further consideration given to the requirements of the Board of Education regarding clinical teaching. A scheme was suggested to the effect that the Infirmary staff should amalgamate with the present Board to form the Board of the Faculty of Medicine. Of this Board, two sub-committees should be formed, one to regulate teaching at the Faculty of Medicine, and the other to regulate clinical teaching which should be composed of the present Infirmary Faculty.'

In addition it was agreed that on the nomination of the Infirmary Faculty the University would appoint a medical and a surgical tutor, each with a salary of £125 per annum. The first were Dr G. W. Watson and Mr Alfred Gough. In the same year, in April 1910, the Board of the Infirmary at last agreed that 'Women students be admitted to the practice of the Infirmary with the exception of the Male Out-patient Department'. This was the end of a long struggle which was considered in the last chapter.

Medical Qualifications

It has been noted that in the early days of the School the qualifications for entry into practice were either Membership of the Royal College of Surgeons of England or the Licence of the Society of Apothecaries. It was some years before most provincial medical students could obtain a degree unless they had been at a university. Recognition of the Liverpool school as qualified to grant certificates of attendance for graduation in the University of London was obtained in 1839. In the same year this was sought, unsuccessfully, by the Leeds school but in 1858 the University of London fully opened its examinations to external students.

The Conjoint Board Examination and Curriculum were derived largely from the new licence of the Royal College of Physicians of London of 1862 though the combination with the Royal College of Surgeons of England did not take place until 1884 and the first examinations were held in January 1885. The qualification LRCP, MRCS largely supplanted the LSA.

Victoria University in Manchester, with Owens College as its only constituent college, received its charter in 1880. University College in Liverpool and the Yorkshire College in Leeds became additional constituent colleges of Victoria University in 1884 and 1887 respectively. From this time students at the Leeds Medical School could graduate MB (Vict) without leaving the city for this examination. From 1904, when the University of Leeds received its charter the students, of course, could graduate MB (Leeds). In addition there were the students who went to Oxford or Cambridge before carrying out their hospital training in Leeds. They usually qualified as BM or MB of their Universities though some were satisfied with the LRCP, MRCS.

It is interesting to note that the total cost of medical education varied somewhat according to the course taken. The Yorkshire College Calendar for 1903–04 summarised this as follows for the degree MB, ChB of Victoria University and for the diplomas MRCS, LRCP of the Conjoint Board:

'VICTORIA UNIVERSITY	£	s	d
Preliminary Scientific Year —	26	0	0
Medical School Composition Fee	67	4	0
Hospital, including Fever Hospital, Obstetric Course, and instruction in Vaccination	48	16	6
University Examinations (three)	15	0	0
	£157	0	6

CONJOINT BOARD —	£	s	d
Preliminary Scientific Year	17	11	0
Medical School Composition Fee	67	4	0
Hospital, including Fever Hospital, Obstetric Course, and instruction in Vaccination	48	16	6
Conjoint Board Examinations (three)	42	0	0
	£175	11	6

In addition to the fees, the sum required for dissection expenses, books, microscope, small apparatus and clinical appliances, together with the subscription to the Students' Union, may be estimated in each case as about £21; and in the case of the London Diploma there are to be added the travelling expenses and maintenance in town during each examination.'

CHAPTER NINE

The Establishment of Chairs and Departments

UNTIL the amalgamation of the Yorkshire College and the Medical School in 1884 the staff of the latter were part-time teachers. The appointment in 1874 of full-time professors of CHEMISTRY, PHYSICS and BIOLOGY in the College solved the problem of the teaching of medical students in the first stage of the curriculum but the teaching of anatomy and physiology in the second remained a problem. As a result a full-time Chair in PHYSIOLOGY was established in 1884 (Professor de Burgh Birch). The Chair of ANATOMY continued to be occupied by a part-time professor. From 1887 this was Dr T. W. Griffith but in 1910 it became full-time and Dr J. K. Jamieson was appointed. A similar state of affairs occurred in the Department of PATHOLOGY where the enthusiastic part-time teaching of Dr Jacob and Dr Trevelyan, physicians at the Infirmary, delayed the establishment of a full-time Chair until 1904 when Professor A. S. Leyton was appointed.

The amalgamation of the Medical School and the Yorkshire College resulted in a part-time Chair of MEDICINE. Dr J. E. Eddison was the first incumbent and the situation remained the same until Dr R. E. Tunbridge (later Sir Ronald) was appointed as full-time professor in 1946.

In SURGERY also there was a part-time professor from 1884 (Mr T. R. Jessop). In 1910 an additional part-time Chair in Clinical Surgery was established with Mr B. G. A. Moynihan (later Lord Moynihan), Jessop's son-in-law, as the first professor. He became professor of Surgery in 1925. A full-time Chair in Surgery was not established until 1954 when Professor John C. Goligher was appointed.

It was reported in May 1899 that a bacteriology class had been formed in the Department of Pathology, one member of which was a woman. Two months later the professor, Dr Trevelyan, stated that several departments of the Yorkshire College namely Chemistry, Agriculture and Tanning desired to include bacteriology in their scheme of instruction. Bacteriology, as mentioned, was included in the Department of Pathology and Professor Trevelyan pointed out in 1900 that there was inadequate accommodation for it, there being no proper laboratory, no room for the preparation of media and no research room. In 1919 Dr J. W. McLeod was appointed to the new lectureship in Bacteriology at the Medical School and as assistant bacteriologist to the Infirmary. He had worked during the war of 1914–18 on trench fever, trench nephritis and dysentery. In 1922 Lord Brotherton of Wakefield endowed a Chair of BACTERIOLOGY and McLeod became the first professor. He continued in this position until 1952 during which period he carried out many important investigations which were recognised by his election to the Fellowship of the Royal Society in 1933. His successor in 1952, Professor C. L. Oakley, also became FRS. In 1973 two Chairs in MICROBIOLOGY were created and Professors D. H. Watson and E. Mary Cooke were appointed.

MATERIA MEDICA AND THERAPEUTICS were taught from the foundation of the School, the first lecturer being Dr Hunter. In 1884 Dr J. B. Hellier held the post and was succeeded in 1889 by Dr A. G. Barrs who became the first Professor (part-time) in these subjects in May 1894.

Ten years later there were discussions on the establishment of a full-time Chair in Pharmacology and Therapeutics. It was thought that the time was not opportune but that the Chair of Materia Medica and Therapeutics, vacant since Dr Barrs became Professor of Medicine in 1898, should not be filled but that a lecturer be appointed. From 1914 to 1926 Mr J. H. Gough was lecturer in Materia Medica and Pharmacy followed by Mr J. J. Anning until about 1936. However, in 1917 Dr Lovatt Evans was appointed Professor of Experimental Physiology and Experimental Pharmacology. A full-time Chair of PHARMACOLOGY was not established until 1946 when Professor W. A. Bain was appointed.

From the foundation of the School MIDWIFERY AND THE DISEASES OF WOMEN AND CHILDREN were taught by Mr Samuel Smith for the next thirty-five years. He lectured at 7 am on Mondays and Thursdays and it was said that he was never late.

In 1884, when the Medical Department of the Yorkshire College began its first session, Dr C. J. Wright lectured on Midwifery and Dr James Braithwaite on Diseases of Women and Children. A professorship of Midwifery (part-time) was created in 1888 and Dr Wright was appointed. It became a Chair of Obstetrics in 1904 with the same incumbent. From 1889 Dr J. B. Hellier was lecturer in Gynaecology and it was not until 1945 that there was a full-time Chair in Obstetrics and Gynaecology occupied by Professor A. M. Claye (later Sir Andrew).

A part-time lectureship on MENTAL DISEASES was established in 1884 and in March Dr Major was appointed with Dr Bevan Lewis of Wakefield to assist him. Dr Major resigned a month later but Dr Bevan Lewis continued in the post. From 1911 there was a part-time Chair in Mental Diseases and Psychiatry held by Professor Shaw Bolton, a distinguished psychiatrist, until 1934. The title of the Chair was changed to that of Psychological Medicine and in 1946 the first full-time Professor, H. V. Dicks, was appointed.

A part-time lectureship in Hygiene was established in 1884 and Mr R. N. Hartley, a surgeon to the Leeds Public Dispensary, was appointed. The title of the department was changed to that of PUBLIC HEALTH in 1896 and again in 1948 to Preventive Medicine and Public Health. After Mr Hartley retired in 1904 a part-time Chair was created which was occupied by the Medical Officer of Health for Leeds. The first incumbent was Dr J. S. Cameron who was succeeded in 1917 by Professor W. Angus for two years, followed by Professor J. J. Jervis. The Department of Community Health and General Practice replaced the Department of Public Health on the retirement of Professor Bradshaw in October 1973.

A part-time lectureship in OPHTHALMOLOGY was instituted in 1884 though it was not until 1911 that the eye and ear surgical practice in the General Infirmary, previously combined, was divided. As a result a part-time lectureship in Otology was instituted in 1912, leading later to the establishment of the EAR, NOSE AND THROAT DEPARTMENT.

A proposal in 1912 to recommend the institution of a lectureship in ANAESTHETICS was rejected by the Board but in January 1920 Dr Douglas Seaton, a general practitioner who had been an anaesthetist to the Infirmary from 1900 and surgeon at the Leeds Public Dispensary from 1903, was appointed honorary lecturer in this subject. The situation as regards the lectureship remained the same, with part-time anaesthetists holding the post, until 1947 when a full-time Reader (Dr R. P. Harbord) was appointed. On his resignation in 1963 a full-time Chair of Anaesthesia was created and in 1964 Dr J. F. Nunn was appointed Professor. He established a distinguished scientific department which carried out much research in a subject that has advanced greatly in the last three decades.

In December 1918 Mr G. Winfield was appointed lecturer in Physiology and Biochemistry, followed by Mr Wormald as Reader in Biochemistry and in 1927 the Professor of Physiology, Dr McSwiney, raised the question of the position of BIOCHEMISTRY in the University, pointing out that the institution of a separate department in this subject in the main buildings at University Road would be injurious to the interests of the Department of Physiology. He urged that resistance should be offered to any attempt to divorce the subject from its functional side. In October 1926 Mr F. C. Happold had been appointed as Demonstrator in the Department of Pathology and Bacteriology and in 1931 he became a Lecturer in Bacteriology. He was working on the biochemistry of bacteria. In 1945 a Chair of Biochemistry was established in the Department of Physiology and he became the first Professor. The autonomous Department of Biochemistry appeared in 1947.

W. C. Roentgen, Professor of Physics of Wurzburg, published his communication on the physical characteristics of X-rays on 28 December 1895. Sometime in 1896 X-ray photographs began to be taken in the General Infirmary at Leeds. This had no impact on the Medical School for a long time. In April 1914 the Board of the Faculty agreed that a course in radiology was undesirable and it was not until ten years later that a lectureship in the subject was instituted. This was entitled a 'Lectureship in Medical Radiology and Electro-Therapeutics' and Dr Scargill and Dr Cooper were appointed joint lecturers, the former being chiefly concerned with diagnostic radiology and the latter with radiotherapy.

Radium was used at the Infirmary as a therapeutic agent from 1903 but only occasionally until 1921 when radium worth £3000 was lent to the Infirmary by the Yorkshire Council of the British Empire Cancer Campaign. Within five months, unfortunately, some of this radium had been lost. A radium department was therefore set up at the Infirmary in 1929. By 1934 the increased use of X-rays and radium required the advice of a physicist. Professor R. Whiddington, FRS, Professor of Physics at the University, was asked to act in an advisory capacity. A few months later the Yorkshire Council of the British Empire Cancer Campaign agreed to make a grant for five years towards the salary of a physicist. In June 1935 Dr F. W. Spiers, who had been working in Professor Whiddington's department, was appointed and when the Chair of MEDICAL PHYSICS was instituted in 1948 he became the first Professor.

Also in 1948 was created a part-time Chair in DIAGNOSTIC RADIOLOGY (Professor A. S. Johnstone). This has since become a full-time Chair, when in 1973 Professor M. S. F. MacLachlan was appointed. The first full-time Professor of RADIOTHERAPY was Professor P. B. Kunkler appointed in 1968.

The Radiotherapy Department is still closely associated with that of Medical Physics. It became a national radiotherapy centre serving, with an associate centre in Hull, the Leeds Region. As the result of the initiative of Sir George Martin a remarkable effort resulted in the Regional High Energy Radiation Centre at Cookridge. The Board of Governors of the United Leeds Hospitals paid £40,000 for the building, the Leeds Regional Hospital Board paid for the alterations, under the direction of Professor (later Sir) F. S. Dainton, FRS, of the Department of Physical Chemistry, Leeds University built the laboratories, the Rockefeller Foundation provided the radioactive cobalt and the council of the British Empire Cancer Campaign bought the containers for it. It is still amongst the most up-to-date centres of radiotherapy in the country.

A new branch of radiology appeared after the Second World War: the use of radioactive isotopes both in diagnosis and treatment, as well as in research. Until the advent of the atomic pile such isotopes were costly and scarce but since 1946 they have become readily accessible. In 1960 the Department of Nuclear Medicine was instituted under the charge of Dr C. J. Hayter, though isotopes were being used in the Infirmary for some years before then.

The Board of the Faculty recommended in April 1912 the creation of a Lectureship in CHEMICAL PHYSIOLOGY. Whether this step was the beginning of the department of CHEMICAL PATHOLOGY is not clear, but Dr H. S. Raper was Lecturer in Chemical Physiology in 1914 in the Department of Physiology. In 1925 Dr F. S. Fowweather was appointed Lecturer in Clinical Chemical Pathology and Reader in 1931. This was in the Department of Pathology and Bacteriology. He was appointed Professor in 1945 when the Chair of Chemical Pathology was created within the same department but the Chair became independent in 1951. Professor Fowweather retired in 1956 and was followed (in 1957) by Professor G. H. Lathe.

In March 1926 the Board of the Faculty recommended the creation of a Chair of Experimental Pathology within the Department of Pathology and Bacteriology, the holder to be Director of CANCER RESEARCH.

Professor R. D. Passey was appointed and occupied the Chair from 1926 to 1953. The department became autonomous in 1951 and was greatly supported by the British Empire Cancer Campaign. In addition to the distinguished work of Professor Passey there was that of Dr Georgiana Bonser and others.

In 1927 a part-time lectureship in DERMATOLOGY was instituted within the Department of Medicine when Dr J. T. Ingram was appointed the first Consultant in Dermatology at the General Infirmary at Leeds. In 1948 the Department of Dermatology became autonomous and in 1950 there were three part-time lecturers.

RHEUMATOLOGY in Leeds began in 1934 when Dr (later Professor) S. J. Hartfall and Dr H. G. Garland opened a special clinic at the Leeds Public Dispensary to treat patients with rheumatoid arthritis by the injection of gold salts. This clinic had become very busy by 1937 and was held twice weekly. In February of that year Dr W. Goldie was appointed as a research worker in the clinic and a month later was appointed by the University as Research Fellow in co-operation with the Royal Bath Hospital in Harrogate. The work was stopped by the Second World War and was not restarted. Goldie became a Lecturer in Pathology at the University in 1946, and the University appointed a director of research in Rheumatology in 1948. In 1964 Dr V. Wright was made Senior Lecturer in the subject and became Professor of Rheumatology in 1970.

The rise in the incidence of venereal diseases during the First World War in both the military and civilian population caused great concern and in 1916 clinics were set up under Local Government Boards throughout the country. At the General Infirmary such a clinic was opened in October 1916 with Dr Vining as Senior Officer in charge and in 1919 Dr Bibby took over. It then became part of the Department of Medicine in the Medical School, but in 1948–49 a part-time lectureship in VENEREOLOGY was established and this was separated from the Department of Medicine.

The Department of NEUROLOGY appeared in 1948 when Dr H. G. Garland was appointed lecturer, and about the same time several departments, previously in the Department of Medicine, became autonomous: INFECTIOUS DISEASES, Venereal Diseases (as mentioned) and TUBERCULOSIS. Also at that time some departments previously within the Department of Surgery separated from it including ORTHOPAEDIC SURGERY, THORACIC SURGERY and NEUROLOGICAL SURGERY. The Departments of PLASTIC SURGERY and PAEDIATRIC SURGERY appeared a little later.

The Department of UROLOGY was created in 1952 with Mr (later Professor) L. N. Pyrah in charge. As a result of Professor Pyrah's efforts a Urology Research Unit was established in the Wellcome Wing of the Infirmary. It was opened in November 1961 and was in part transformed into the Medical Research Council's MINERAL METABOLISM UNIT within the University in September 1964 with Dr (later Professor) B. E. C. Nordin in charge. The Urology Research Unit continued under Dr F. M. Parsons.

A part-time lectureship in MEDICAL GENETICS was established in 1951 but this was replaced by a full-time lectureship in Genetics in the Faculty of Science in October 1962 and a Chair in this subject was created in 1966.

The Department of IMMUNOLOGY was instituted by the University in 1966 but it was not until 1969 that Professor G. Gowland became the first occupant of the Chair.

St James's Hospital became a University of Leeds Teaching Hospital and the first appointment was that of Professor M. S. Losowsky to the Chair of Medicine in May 1969. He took up his duties in the following October. Other departments were created: in 1973 Professor G. R. Giles was appointed to the Chair of Surgery and in the same year Professor D. C. A. Bevis to the Chair of Obstetrics and Gynaecology.

In 1979 the Department of Psychiatry was instituted with Professor A. C. P. Sims in the Chair, that of Paediatrics and Child Health in 1980 (Professor S. R. Meadow) and that of Orthopaedic Surgery (Professor R. A. Dickson) in 1981. There is also a Medical Physics Unit of the University at the hospital.

CHAPTER TEN

Dental School and Further Building

THE RECOGNITION of dental surgery in Leeds began in February 1881 when Mr T. S. Carter was elected honorary dental surgeon to the General Infirmary. In November of the same year Mr G. A. C. Benham was appointed to a similar position at the Leeds Public Dispensary.

In December 1888 the Dean read a 'Memorial presented by a Committee appointed by the Dentists of the town praying for the establishment of a complete Dental Curriculum in connexion with the Medical Department of the Yorkshire College'.[1] The Dean read an extract (dated 1882) from the minutes of the late School of Medicine showing that the subject had then been under consideration.[2] The matter was deferred.

However, the question continued to be discussed and in 1900, when the new Public Dispensary was being planned, the idea of a dental hospital in Leeds had the support of the Infirmary Board and the Yorkshire College. In May 1900 the Faculty of the Dispensary adopted the following resolution: 'That the Dispensary Committee be urged to start a Dental Department to co-operate with the Medical Department of the Yorkshire College, & with the Infirmary, in providing a complete course in Dentistry in Leeds'. This was accepted and the Planning Committee for the new Dispensary were instructed to include five rooms for the accommodation of a Dental Department. The intention was that no lectures would be given at the Dispensary, the work there being purely clinical. The lectures would be given at the Yorkshire College. The students at the Dispensary would not only receive instruction but would help with the work of the Department. There was some opposition to the scheme but in February 1902 the Committee of the Dispensary agreed to proceed with it.

In April 1904 the administrative details were laid down and in January 1905 the honorary dental surgeons: six surgeons and six assistant dental

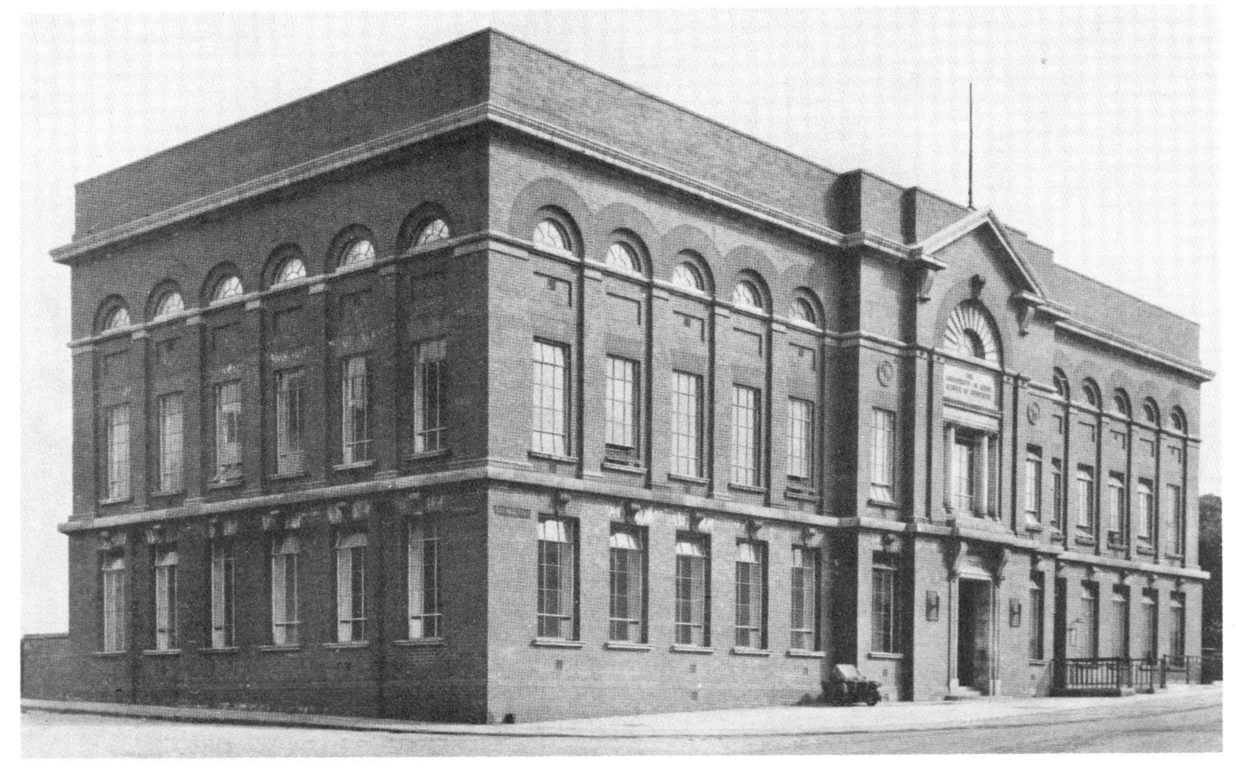

FIG. 28 *Dental School and Hospital, 1928*

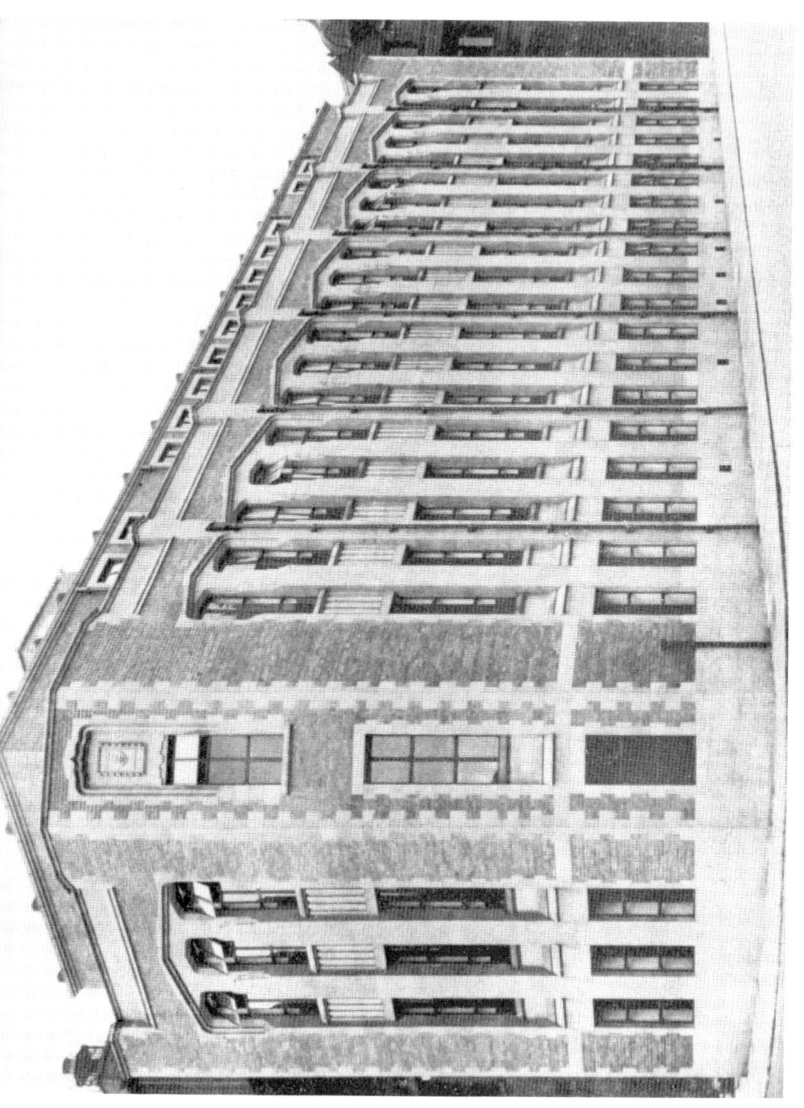

FIG. 29 *Physiology Extension (west wing of Thoresby Place School), 1930*

surgeons, were elected. Three honorary anaesthetists were also appointed.

In 1906 the Dental Hospital was recognised by the University of Leeds and by the Royal College of Surgeons of England as a school where students taking the course for the Diploma in Dental Surgery could undertake the necessary clinical practice and receive training in dental mechanics. An agreement between the University and the Dispensary bringing the teaching at the Dental Department of the Leeds Public Dispensary into the University was reached in 1914 and this is when the University Dental School, as distinct from the Dental Hospital, came into being. However, between 1906 and 1914 individual members of the staff of the Dental Hospital had been appointed University lecturers to give the formal teaching required by students taking the LDS course and examinations. The first of the students to qualify was Harold R. Bentley who was awarded the LDS (Leeds) in June 1910.

In December 1912 the Warden of the Dental Department (Mr Stephen D. Hey) wrote to the Committee of the Dispensary that the rooms at the disposal of the Department were inadequate on account of the increase in the work carried out. The Dental Committee thought it probable that some arrangements might be made with the Board of the General Infirmary in connection with their extension scheme, to provide a more suitable home for the work. In May 1913 there were discussions about an appeal to the public for funds to build a dental hospital on a site offered by the Board of the Infirmary. The matter continued to be discussed at intervals but, no doubt owing to the World War 1914–18 nothing was achieved.

The next development was in May 1920 when the Board of the Infirmary agreed to lend to the University School of Dentistry 'a portion of the old Out-patient Waiting Hall and one of the Theatres and three attendant rooms at the head of the grand staircase'. The move took place about October 1920 and it was not until March 1928 that a new Dental School and Hospital, built on Infirmary land and adjacent to it, was opened (Fig 28).

At the Dispensary dental treatment continued with one honorary dental surgeon. In October 1920 Mr J Kenneth Crawford was elected and he remained until 1923 but in 1927 dental treatment ceased there.

A full-time Chair in Dental Surgery was established in 1931 and Professor Talmage Read was the first to occupy it.

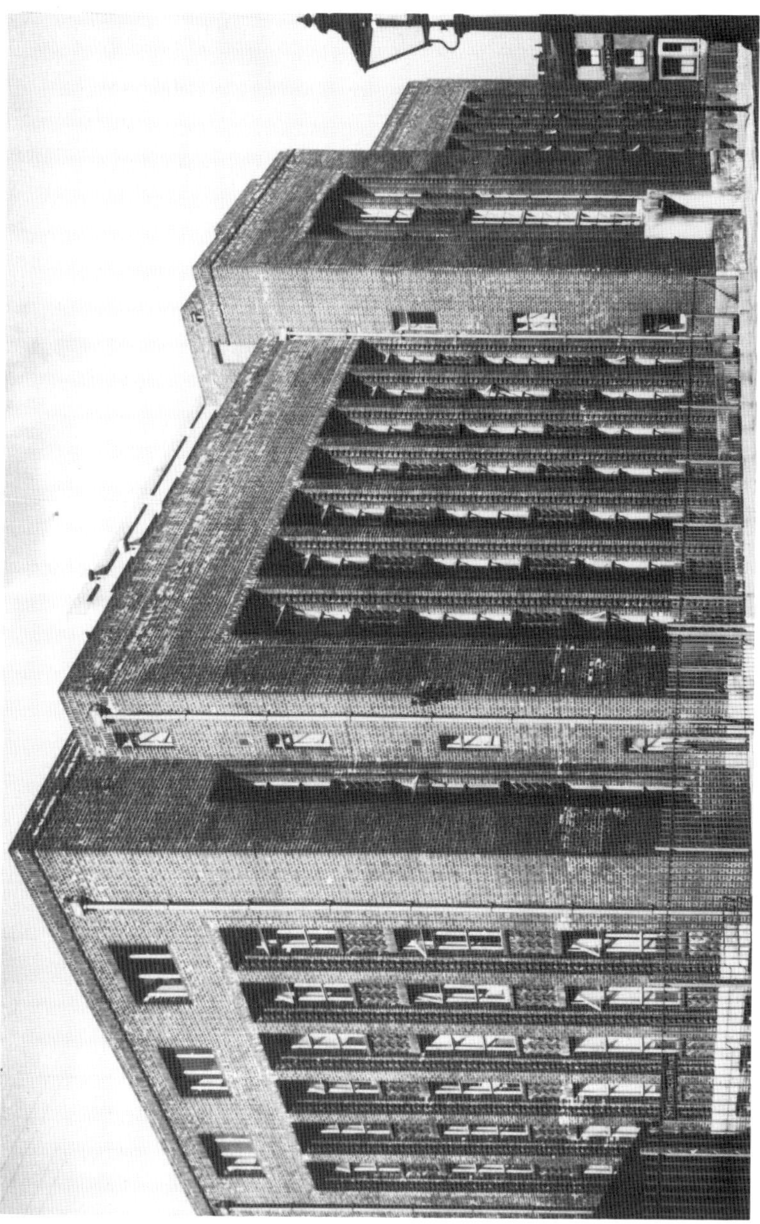

FIG. 30 *Algernon Firth Institute of Pathology, 1933*

Further Building

In 1904 the recurring problem of inadequate accommodation was raised in regard to the Department of Pathology. Nothing was achieved though the necessity of extensions was again urged in 1912 and 1913. But then came World War One (1914–18) and it was not until 1925 that the matter was brought up again. Pathology and bacteriology had expanded rapidly and the entrance of women students (see pp 96, 98) was another unexpected development causing shortage of space.

When Professor McSwiney came to the Chair of Physiology in 1926 he found the accommodation of the department inadequate for the growing needs of teaching and research but, with the support of the Dean, Professor Jamieson, he obtained a new wing which was opened in 1930 (Fig 29). The Departments of Pathology and Bacteriology had to wait longer. In 1922 Lord Brotherton endowed a Chair of Bacteriology and Professor Walter McLeod was the first to occupy it. He and his staff had to manage in cramped conditions in St George's House close to the Medical School until the Algernon Firth Institute, designed by John Proctor, FRIBA, was opened in 1933 to house the Departments of Pathology, Bacteriology and Cancer Research (Fig 30).

REFERENCES

1. Yorkshire College, Medical Department Minute Book, 6 December 1888.
2. Leeds School of Medicine Council Book 4, 16 June 1882.

CHAPTER ELEVEN

Some Outstanding Deans

THOMAS SCATTERGOOD

Thomas Scattergood was born in Huddersfield in 1826, the son of the Rev T. Scattergood. Nothing is known of his early life but in August 1846, with four others, he applied for the post of assistant apothecary at the General Infirmary at Leeds and was successful. He was described in the Infirmary minute book as 'from Newcastle'. At that time his aunt, Miss Sarah Page, was matron at the Infirmary — she held the appointment from 1826 until her death in 1852.

Scattergood continued as assistant apothecary until October 1850 about which time he qualified as MRCS and LSA. He had been granted three weeks' leave in August, probably to enable him to take the examinations. It was early in 1851 that he went into general practice in Leeds, in Hunslet Road, and from a letter written by his father we learn that in the first nine months he earned £23. He also worked as an analytical chemist.

His connection with the Leeds School of Medicine began in 1845 as a student and continued for fifty-five years. In 1851 he became Lecturer in Chemistry and from 1869 until June 1888 Lecturer in Forensic Medicine and Toxicology. His medico-legal case books (two volumes in the Medical School Library) have been described by M. A. Green (1973).[1]

On 31 May 1854 Scattergood married Miss Haigh, the daughter of William Haigh, accountant of Leeds, and Mary, née Page. They had six children, three of whom were sons. One, Arthur Kimberley, practised medicine in Blenheim Square, Leeds, and another, Oliver, in Settle.

Some general practitioners in those days developed special interests and on account of this Scattergood was appointed honorary surgeon to the Hospital for Women and Children in 1863 and continued so until he became consultant surgeon in 1889.

An important achievement of Scattergood was the work he did leading to the amalgamation of the Medical School with the Yorkshire College

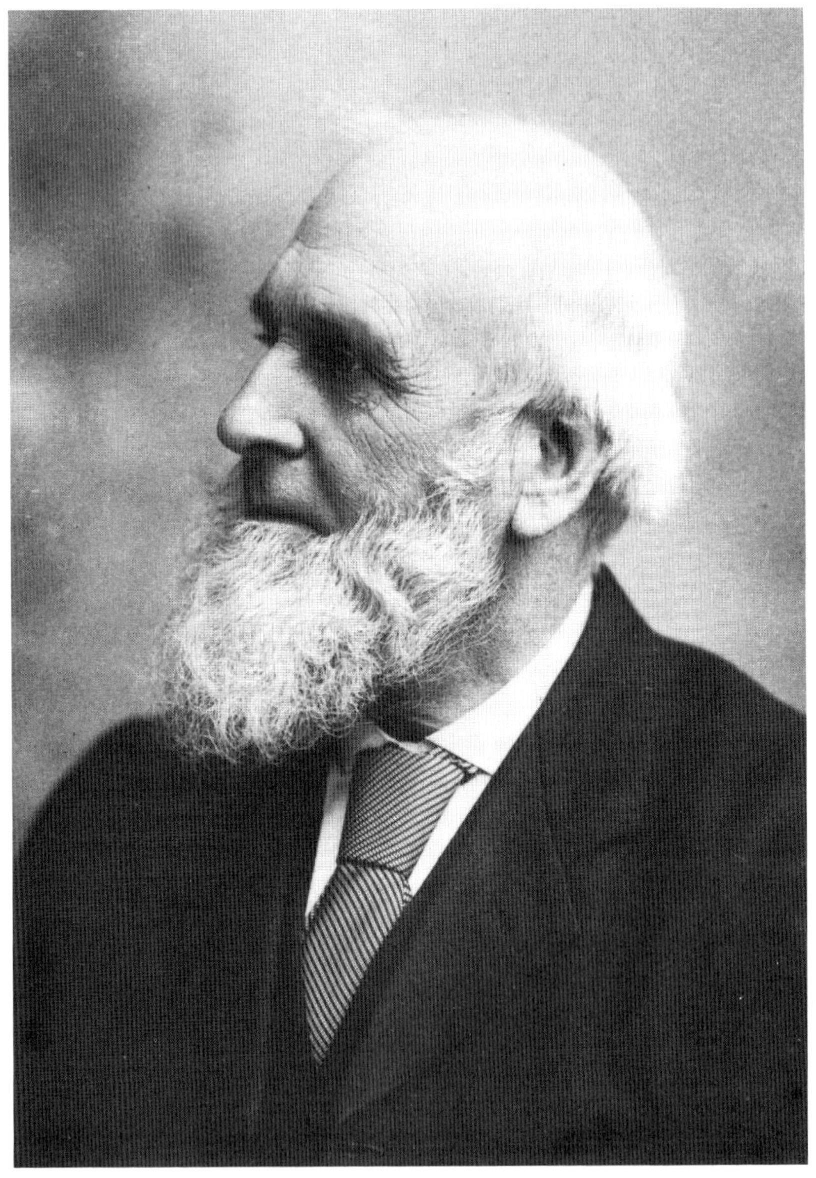

FIG. 31 *Thomas Scattergood*

which had been founded in 1874. After much discussion this union took place in 1884 and the Leeds Medical School became the Faculty of Medicine at the Yorkshire College with Scattergood as Dean, an appointment he held until his death.

He died in February 1900 at 41 Park Square. It is not clear how long this had been his home and where he practised but he was certainly there in 1888.

From the Minute of the Medical Department of 23 February 1900 we read that '. . . It was indeed fortunate for the School of Medicine that at a most critical period in its history it had the devoted services of one who was so peculiarly fitted for the position which he held. His discretion, tact & clearness of vision were invaluable in the negotiations which led to the union of the School with the College. His activity & success in raising funds for the endowment of the Chair of Physiology enabled the Department of Medicine to enter upon its new career with an important improvement of the staff. And a few years later his enthusiasm, his faith in the future, and his firm determination to better the conditions of medical education mainly led to the rebuilding of the School. . . .'

The Council of the Yorkshire College unanimously adopted the following resolution with regard to the services of the late Mr Scattergood:

'He took part in the foundation of the College, was an active member of its Council from the commencement, and in every possible way showed his sincere interest in the work of the institution.

'While every branch of liberal education had his warm support, his chief concern was undoubtedly centred in the department of medicine which he served with an ardour which would have appeared extraordinary even in the case of a man of leisure, with but few other public interests, and was truly remarkable as evinced in the life of Mr Scattergood, with the daily responsibilities of a large practice, and with his active connection with so many other institutions for the cultivation of those moral and intellectual forces that tend to the highest welfare of the community. The present Medical School is to a great extent a monument to Mr Scattergood, to whose energy and persistent advocacy the new building is in great measure due. As Dean of the Medical Department from the union of the Leeds School of Medicine with the Yorkshire College up to the time of his death, he has left a record of devotion which will remain as a stimulus to his former colleagues, and an example of what is possible to those who follow him. . . .'

From the Minutes of the Medical Department we learn that the secretaries of the Scattergood portrait fund, which paid for the portrait of him which hangs in the Medical School, handed over to the Faculty £140 for a Scattergood Prize in Obstetrics and Gynaecology which is still awarded annually.

JOHN KAY JAMIESON, MB, CM Edin (1894), LLD Leeds (1936), MA Dublin (1938), MCh Dublin (1947)[2]

J. K. Jamieson, known to all his friends, acquaintances and students as 'Jimmy', or 'Jamie' or 'J.K.', was born in July 1873, the fourth son of Robert Jamieson of Sandness and his wife Barbara (née Laing). Several other children of this marriage distinguished themselves academically. He attended the Sandness Madras School which his father had established before the Scottish Education Act of 1872 with the assistance, it is understood, of the trustees of the Rev Dr Andrew Bell (1753–1832), himself the founder of the Madras College at St Andrews. J.K. and his five brothers, in their turn, served the school as pupil-teachers. Their father was not only founder and schoolmaster but also local postmaster, session clerk and emigration agent.

From this school he and his brothers went on to the University of Edinburgh and J.K. graduated MB, CM in 1894. His first six months after qualification were spent as demonstrator of anatomy in the School of Medicine of the Royal Colleges at Surgeons' Hall, Edinburgh, under Macdonald Brown. In April 1895 he came to Leeds as demonstrator of anatomy under Professor Thomas Wardrop Griffith, a post which he held for fifteen years. In June 1904 his salary was raised from £100 to £200 per annum. In 1910, on Griffith's translation to the Chair of Medicine, Jamieson was appointed the first whole-time Professor of Anatomy in the Leeds School. In those early days, with no administrative duties outside the Department of Anatomy, he had both the time and the opportunity for teaching and of these he took full advantage. His views on the teaching of anatomy to medical students were eminently sane and sensible: he was convinced that a sound training in human anatomy was the only true basis for clinical work. A teacher of the first

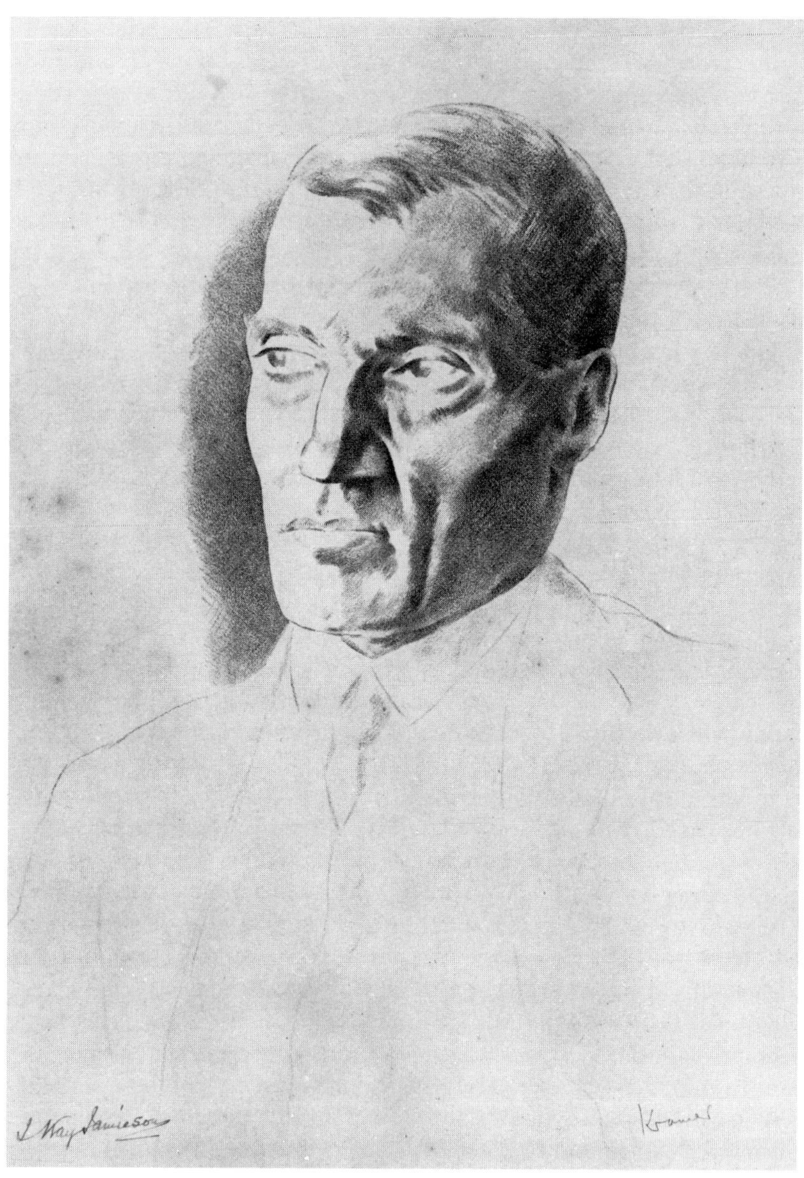

FIG. 32 *John Kay Jamieson, lithograph by Jacob Kramer*

rank, he had as demonstrator been a tower of strength to the School. Later, when other interests claimed much of his time, he continued to devote some hours of nearly every day to lecturing and to dissecting-room teaching. His blackboard drawings were superb and he could draw a perfect circle standing sideways to the blackboard, swinging his arm round at the shoulder. He could draw a symmetrical thorax using both hands at the same time. Though a lucid and stimulating lecturer it was in the dissecting-room that he showed to fullest advantage. Nor was his teaching merely morphological: with him structure and function always went hand in hand and were always integrated.

On 18 October 1906 Jamieson married Elisabeth, daughter of R. P. Goodworth of Winterton in Lincolnshire. They had two children: Barbara J. Jamieson, MBE, BSc (Lond), formerly dietician to the Royal Masonic Hospital, London, who gave up the post to keep house for her father in Dublin, and Dr John Jamieson who, after a period of great hardship as prisoner of war in Greece and Germany, was Senior School Medical Officer in Leeds.

Jamieson numbered among the firm friends of his demonstratorship period both Moynihan and Dobson. It was with Dobson that he collaborated in the work on the surgical anatomy of the lymphatic system, particularly of the tongue, stomach and large intestine, which is his chief claim to fame as an anatomical investigator. Their work, published in the years 1907–20, has stood the test of time and is now part of the *corpus* of anatomical knowledge.

It was during the First World War that Jamieson got the opportunity of showing that in addition to being a supremely good teacher he was also a most able administrator. De Burgh Birch, Professor of Physiology and, during most of his tenure of the chair, the only whole-time professor in the Medical School, had been Dean of the Faculty of Medicine from 1900 to 1906. In 1913 he had commenced a second tour of duty in this office. On the outbreak of war in 1914 he was mobilised as a Colonel of Territorials and left Leeds (he had formed the Leeds Company Volunteer Medical Staff Corps at the School in 1896). Jamieson was appointed Acting Dean, a post which he held for three years. He had already, since 1910, been Sub-Dean of the Faculty and, during the same period resident Warden of Lyddon Hall, then the only men's hostel in the University. In March 1915 he was commissioned as Major and appointed registrar of the East Leeds War Hospital in Beckett

Street, of which, together with the 2nd Northern General Hospital at Beckett Park, Harry Littlewood, formerly senior surgeon to the General Infirmary at Leeds and Professor of Surgery, was commanding officer. During the course of the war both these hospitals were very greatly expanded, and in 1917 Jamieson was promoted Lieutenant-Colonel and became administrator of his hospital. The onerous duties of this post he carried out with the greatest efficiency, while continuing also to give part of his time to undergraduate teaching. Jamieson took the keenest interest in the welfare of the members of staff of the East Leeds War Hospital, especially the non-commissioned officers and men, all of whom held him in high regard. After the war he was a warm supporter of the annual reunions of the men of the unit, and rarely failed to take the chair on these occasions.

He was elected Dean of the Faculty of Medicine and chairman of its Board in 1918, before he had completed his Army service. These complementary offices he held for the record period of eighteen years. As we have seen, the first Dean of the Faculty of Medicine after the amalgamation with the Yorkshire College was Thomas Scattergood who served in that capacity from 1884 until 1900. It was Jamieson's ambition to beat that record, and he did so by two years. During the eighteen years between 1918 and 1936 he was not merely Dean of the Faculty but also the dominant personality in the School of Medicine. He loved his position of undisputed authority though he held the reins of control lightly and was never given to 'throwing his weight about'. Within the higher administrative bodies of the University he was also a power in the land. During the whole term of his Deanship he was the elected representative of the Faculty of Medicine on the University Council and for most of that time a member also of the Finance Committee, Salaries Committee and House and Estates Committee. In all these important bodies he was valued for his sage and disinterested advice and sound common sense. He was Pro-Vice-Chancellor from 1923 to 1925, and, as there was a long interregnum in the Vice-Chancellorship following the retirement of Sir Michael Sadler in 1923, he served as Acting Vice-Chancellor for the whole of the 1923–24 session.

But it was within his own faculty that he made his most notable contribution to University advancement. He was the mainspring in the important extensions of the School of Medicine which took place between the First and Second World Wars. The School of Dentistry was provided with a fine new building, opened in 1928, which admirably served the dual purpose of Dental School and Hospital (Fig 28). Large extensions to the Department of Physiology followed, and were opened in 1930, paving the way for the subsequent establishment of Departments and Chairs of Biochemistry and Pharmacology.

Next came the building of the Algernon Firth Institute of Pathology. This most necessary addition to the resources of the School of Medicine ran a great risk of being held up indefinitely. So much of the development fund had been lavished on the new Physiology block that not enough was left to erect and equip a building large enough to accommodate both Pathology and Bacteriology. At one time it seemed likely that it would be possible only to equip one or two floors instead of the five considered necessary. It was then that the generosity of Sir Algernon Firth with his gift of £25,000 'towards the building of a pathological institute' made the scheme possible. To Jamieson rightly belongs a large share of the credit for getting this institute established.

In 1936 Mrs Jamieson died and soon after, when within two years of retirement, he was offered and accepted the Chair of Anatomy and Embryology in Trinity College, Dublin in succession to Professor A. F. Dixon. Probably his wife's death influenced him in making this decision. It was to be a seven-year tenure, carrying him on until the age of seventy. When that time arrived there was the Second World War and Jamieson continued in office from year to year. Indeed he carried on the duties of the Chair, though in the face of increasing physical disability, until December 1947. In Dublin he met with the warmest acceptance, both academically and socially. Immediately he felt at home, as well among the Fellows of Trinity as in medical circles. He was duly elected a fellow of the Royal Academy of Medicine in Ireland (later serving as President of the Section of Anatomy and Physiology) and Honorary Anatomist to Sir Patrick Dun's Hospital. He was proud of the fact that his Chair carried with it the additional and ancient title of Professor of Anatomy and Chirurgery. He was no stranger to Dublin. For many years he had been an external examiner in Trinity College, including the period of the First World War and the time of 'the Troubles'. Jamieson had also been external examiner for the Universities of Edinburgh, Aberdeen, Liverpool, Manchester, Sheffield, Bristol, and Belfast. He was elected a Member of the Royal Irish Academy in 1937.

Of the Dublin period Professor J. W. Bigger wrote: 'it would not have been easy for anyone to maintain the reputation of a department of anatomy which had had at its head three such men as Alexander Macalister, D. J. Cunningham, and A. F. Dixon, but we asked Jamieson to do something more difficult than that, to break the tradition of the department. Dixon had maintained, unaltered, the Edinburgh tradition which he had inherited from Cunningham, a tradition which was excellent when medical students were given training in little except anatomy in preparation for their clinical work but a tradition which, in the opinion of the younger members of the staff of the school, had outlived its utility. So it fell to Jamieson to reduce the duration of formal teaching in anatomy from eight terms to five and to prove that, while a course of this length might be inadequate for the training of an anatomist, it was adequate for 99 per cent of medical students. . . .'[3]

Jamieson's services received recognition from both the institutions he had served so well. Leeds made him an honorary LLD in 1937, Trinity accorded him the degrees of MA and MCh *de jure*. His portrait, painted on the commission of his Leeds colleagues by Mr Lee Whelan is now to be found by the Dean's Office in the Leeds Medical School, where it has for companion that of Thomas Scattergood.

The external activities of Jamieson during the Leeds period of his career were numerous and varied. For eight years (1928–36) he represented the University on the General Medical Council. He was an honorary life member of the Leeds and West Riding Medico-Chirurgical Society. He became a Freemason soon after the 1914–18 War and took the duties and responsibilities of the craft very seriously, reaching the grade of Senior Warden in 1929. He would not accept further promotion because of his inability to give the necessary time to the work. A member of Alwoodley Golf Club for many years, he played regularly at weekends and in vacation. When he went to Dublin he joined the Island Golf Club and continued to play a vigorous game until failing health led to curtailment of such activities. For many years he was a governor of Leeds Grammar School and of Leeds Girls' High School.

All his life he was intensely proud of his Norse blood and woe betide anyone who mistook him for a Scot. He died at his home in Black Rock, Co Dublin, on 20 August 1948, eight months after his retirement at the age of seventy-five.

MATTHEW JOHN STEWART, CBE, MB, ChB Glasgow (1907), FRCP London (1924), FRFPS (1932), Hon LLD Glasgow (1938), Hon MD Melbourne (1951)

'Matt' Stewart, a much loved figure in Leeds, was born on 4 May 1885 in Dalmellington, Ayrshire, the son of William Ritchie Stewart, a grocer, who was elected a fellow of the Society of Antiquaries of Scotland for his work on local history and folklore, and Mary McKie, the daughter of a shepherd. He was educated at the local school and at the University of Glasgow where he was Brunton memorial prizeman as the most distinguished graduate of his year. He was then twenty-two and had time to decide in which branch of medicine to practice. While at Ruehill Fever Hospital under Samson Gemmell he learned the value of statistical methods from John Brownlee before working on pathology with J. H. Teacher. He had already come under the influence of Professor Robert Muir who trained so many who were to become important pathologists.

He decided to become a pathologist and in 1910 came to Leeds as clinical pathologist to the General Infirmary. In March 1912 he was appointed Honorary Demonstrator in Clinical Pathology at the Medical School. In 1913 he married Dr Clara Eglington (later OBE), also a pathologist, the daughter of Edward Eglington, a manufacturer in Lichfield. They had no children.

During the war of 1914–18 Stewart was pathologist to the East Leeds War Hospital and later to the 59th General Hospital at St Omer in Northern France. He was recalled in 1918 to fill the Chair of Pathology in Leeds which was vacant as the result of Professor Leyton's retirement in 1917. He resigned from his post at the Infirmary but was appointed physician in pathology. The University Department of Pathology was small at that time but, as we have seen, Professor Stewart, with the active co-operation of Professor J. K. Jamieson, the Dean, soon created within it Chairs of Bacteriology and Cancer Research.

Stewart was a forceful lecturer and a good teacher at all times but as a post-mortem demonstrator he was brilliant. His remarkable powers of observation combined with an unusually retentive memory and much experience in morbid anatomy made his autopsy sessions an experience no student could forget. He also made his department a Mecca for postgraduate students of pathology.

His scientific work was based more on observation than experimentation. He combined with Sir Arthur Hurst to write a standard monograph on peptic ulcer. He also wrote on cellular foreign-body reactions, cholesterin deposits, mycloid tumours in tendon sheaths, chordoma, liver damage in munition workers, asbestosis, siderosis, and silicosis. In particular he is remembered as editor-in-chief of the *Journal of Pathology and Bacteriology* from 1934.

Apart from his work in his own department, he did much for the University. He was academic Sub-Dean in the Faculty of Medicine and then from 1941 to 1948 he was Dean. He had been Pro-Vice-Chancellor from 1939 to 1941 and from 1942 to 1958 he represented the University on the General Medical Council. He also served on the Medical Research Council, doing especially good work for the Arsenic Committee and the Committee on Industrial Pulmonary Disease. These by no means end his contributions for he was on the Pathological Advisory Committee of the National Radium Commission, the histological panel of the British Empire Cancer Campaign and he gave valuable advice as a trustee of the Hunterian Collection of the Royal College of Surgeons of England.

This indefatigable man was also external examiner to the Universities of Oxford, Cambridge, St Andrews, Wales, and Belfast, to the Conjoint Board and to the Faculty of Radiologists. Moreover, he travelled extensively: in Ceylon, Africa, New Zealand, Australia, America, and Jamaica.

Although a strict disciplinarian he was retiring, kindly and had a keen sense of humour. He was a connoisseur of wine and a lover of congenial company. His command of English in the accent of a Scot was superb and he was most knowledgeable about Burns, Pepys and the Brontës. He was a member of the council of the Brontë Society and delighted to be a member of the Pepys Society. At Melbourne in 1951 he gave the Bancroft oration, the title being 'Medicine in Pepys' Diary'. He had many hobbies which included walking, especially in the Yorkshire Dales, literature, church architecture, and philately.

This remarkable man died on 7 November 1956, aged seventy-one, at the home to which he and his wife had retired in Stoke Poges, Buckinghamshire.

REFERENCES

1. M. A. Green, 'Dr Scattergood's Case Books', *The Practitioner*, vol 211, November 1973, pp 679–84.
2. M. J. Stewart, *University of Leeds Review*, 1948–49, 1, p 125 and *Journal of Anatomy*, vol 83, part 1, 1949, p 47.
3. J. W. Bigger, *Lancet*, 1948, ii, p 397.

CHAPTER TWELVE

A Time of Expansion

IN THE LATE NINETEEN FIFTIES the intake of medical students declined to about sixty per year and following the publication of the Willink Report,[1] which had suggested that too many doctors were being trained, it reached the low figure of fifty-three in 1959. However, by this time it was expected that applications would rise again within the next five years to fill all of the eighty places available. In the late 'fifties also, overflows from existing departments, and some new ones were occupying makeshift accommodation in old property near the campus, for example Biochemistry, Paediatrics, Psychiatry, Anaesthetics, Obstetrics, Preventive Medicine, Forensic Medicine, and Oral Biology were housed in this way. Rebuilding of the Leeds General Infirmary was being considered, the centre of the town was being actively redeveloped, including the planning of an inner ring road, and the University was expanding rapidly (from roughly 3200 students in 1953 to 4600 in 1959). Moreover it was known that the increased birth-rate following the end of World War Two had produced a 'bulge' which would reach university entrance in the middle 'sixties.

Rather than allow uncontrolled expansion and building in a haphazard fashion, the University had invited in 1958 Mr Peter Chamberlin of Chamberlin, Powell and Bon, architects, to consider how the University should develop over the next decade. Mr Chamberlin acted on the assumption that student numbers would grow to 5500 by 1965 and perhaps to 7000 by 1970 and that 'no definite end to the developmental problem could be foreseen'.

The Chamberlin Development Plan was published in 1960. The plan was comprehensive and imaginative. It noted the sloping nature of the site, the area being proposed for slum clearance, with the sewers, gas mains and electric cables associated with it. It advocated that a larger site area extending as far as Clarendon Road be reserved for University and hospitals. It emphasised the importance of planning a new Teaching

Hospital, Medical School and School of Dentistry at one and the same time if they were to be closely and sympathetically integrated — 'it is vitally important to reach agreement in principle about whether or not a new Teaching Hospital should be built before any planning of the new Medical School is started' and it strongly recommended the covering of the Inner Ring Road so that the road would not divide the total University/Hospital site into two parts.[2]

Though other suggestions that the hospital be developed on new ground to the north west of the medical school and have some single-storey buildings interspersed with patios were not followed, the main cue was taken and the Board of Governors of the United Leeds Hospitals sought agreement in principle from the Ministry of Health for a new Teaching Hospital. Agreement was confirmed in 'A Hospital Plan for England and Wales' published in January 1962[3] and in May 1962 the Board of Governors and the University Council appointed Mr G. Grenfell Baines and Associates of Building Design Partnership as Architects for the joint venture.[4] Co-operation between the Board of Governors and the University over the planning was ensured by the setting up of two bodies, a Joint Planning Committee and a Planning Team. The PLANNING COMMITTEE would deal with policy and had the following membership:

Sir Donald Kaberry (Chairman of the Board of Governors, the United Leeds Hospitals), Sir Charles Morris (Vice-Chancellor), Dr S. T. Anning (Secretary of the Faculty, United Leeds Hospitals), Mr A. B. Pain (Dean, Faculty of Medicine, University of Leeds), Mr J. W. Booth, Professor S. J. Hartfall, Professor C. L. Oakley and Mr W. W. Powell, with Mr J. A. Tunstall (Secretary to the Board, United Leeds Hospitals) and Mr E. W. Williamson (Bursar, The University).

The main functions of the PLANNING TEAM were to co-ordinate information received from hospital and University departments and to provide a brief for the architects. Its members were four administrators devoting their whole time to the work, Mr J. T. Dann, Mr T. McGee, Mr R. E. Jefford, and Miss M. I. McCutcheon (formerly a nursing sister), and three academic members who would devote up to half their time to the team: Professor D. R. Wood, Professor of Pharmacology, nominated by the University Council; Dr D. Taverner, Consultant Physician and Reader in Medicine; and Mr F. G.

Smiddy, Consultant Surgeon and Clinical Lecturer in Surgery, nominated by the University Board of Medicine.[5]

The aim at this stage was to design a Medical Centre, ie a new Teaching Hospital, new Medical School and new Dental School and Hospital to serve the needs of the community and to provide facilities for training 100 medical students and 60 dental students per year. An early report on the proposed bed complement of the hospital added 'And it is fundamental to the concept that this training should be carried out in a Medical Centre unified on one site'.[6]

In February 1965 at a Public Enquiry at the Civic Hall proposals were heard for altering the City's 1955 Development Plan to include in the University and Hospital zones land as far west as Clarendon Road; Dr Taverner and Mr Grenfell Baines gave evidence on hospital and medical teaching developments and Mr Williamson and Mr Chamberlin on the overall requirements of the University. There was only one objection to the re-zoning of the land for hospital purposes and the total area available for the Medical Centre became about 43 acres.[7]

The architects were actively engaged from the start and with the planning team set out to discover how departments functioned. There was much discussion with 'the clients' and the work of the first three years culminated in the publication in September 1965 of a hardback report of some 160 pages with numerous illustrations known affectionately as 'the grey book'.[3]

In the meantime in 1962 initial moves were made for the appointment of a Postgraduate Dean, reflecting the importance now being attached to postgraduate training and refresher courses for general practitioners.[8] Dr J. B. Lynch was appointed in May 1964. He moved into rooms on the east side of the Instructional Block of the General Infirmary which were to be his academic home for the next twenty years.

The question had arisen early in 1963 as to whether or not multidiscipline laboratories should be provided. In May Professor Hopper and Dr Newman described their experiences in the USA of the working of these laboratories.[9] Mr Pain visited New York, Harvard, Western Reserve, Stanford, Los Angeles, and Kentucky to see them.[10] Essentially a multidiscipline laboratory provides the student with all the laboratory facilities he requires for one year of his course, a high bench for biochemistry and certain experiments in physiology and pharmacology and a low bench where microscopical work in histology, pathology and microbiology can be done. The low bench can also serve as a study area, with book shelf, lockable cupboard, etc, although a study cubicle was sometimes provided elsewhere, eg near a library. In one school even a dissecting table had intruded into the laboratory.

Here was an exciting new development in medical teaching. Newcastle was to provide them. Should Leeds follow? Their main advantage is that the student is provided with a home base — a bench and locker of his own and this could be available to be used in the evening or throughout the twenty-four hours if local conditions permit. Of course he tends to have less contact with individual departments and if he happens to be in a corner far away from a window he may well be there for the year. Account was also taken of relative costs, since departments with science students need to have departmental laboratories in any case. The matter was felt to be of such importance that Professor D. R. Wood was asked to go to America to investigate the laboratories in use. He visited four centres in September 1963 and reported to a meeting of the Board of Medicine on 7 October summarising his views as to advantages and disadvantages. Everyone knew that the decision once taken would be difficult to reverse on account of its immediate implications for the rest of the planning. 'On a vote, the Board was divided eleven — eleven with eight abstentions and with the Chairman's casting vote it was resolved

> . . . (a) That a separate dissecting room be provided
> (b) That all other laboratory work including embryology and histology be conducted in multidiscipline laboratories. . . .'[11]

So it was that the MDLs were conceived. Some of the other anticipations of the Board that day did not materialise, for example that the units should accommodate not more than sixteen students — in fact they became twenty-four; that laboratories would be required for the first three years of the course and that one laboratory should be shared by fourth-and fifth-year students — in fact they were provided for only the first two years, which is a pity for it has introduced an unfortunate rigidity into the curriculum.

MDLs tend to be as good as the people running them. That they have run so acceptably in Leeds is due to devotion and attention to detail on the part of the technical staff and in no small measure to the late Dr Julia Fourman who as their Director for the first four years of their function both enjoyed and rose to the challenge they presented and also cared passionately for the welfare of the individual student.

At about the same time, June 1963, as decisions on the MDLs were being taken, the Board of Medicine's long-term Curriculum Committee was looking at various options:

1. a three-year preclinical course leading to a BSc, as proposed in a memorandum prepared by Professor Tunbridge and Dr J. A. Sharp;
2. a scheme for an integrated curriculum devised by Professor Lathe, Dr R. P. Hullin and Professor Scott;
3. a combination of (1) and (2); and
4. a memorandum from Professor Oakley suggesting no radical changes in the course but a reconsideration of the examination system.

There was agreement that the scientific content should be increased, that further study concerning the BSc option would be needed, that further integration was necessary but disagreement as to whether this should be 'horizontal', between say preclinical subjects or 'vertical', between basic medical sciences and clinical subjects.

Irrespective of the final outcome however provision for three years of laboratory work should be made and the Board recommended to the Planning Team accordingly.[12]

The first moves were being made at this time for the setting up of a University Television Service.[12] Within six months the Faculty of Medicine had purchased two mobile TV cameras, control units and monitors with four 23 in television receivers at a cost of £2800, and recommended to the Board of Governors that endoscopic equipment be purchased and that cable links should be provided in the Infirmary between X-ray, Medical Physics, operating theatres and Littlewood Hall.[13]

The complicated procedures for authorising the clearance of slum property to make way for the Ring Road underpass had been accomplished by the City in 1962.[14] Demolition of property bordering the network of roads lying between the Medical School and the University began in 1963, the roads themselves disappearing by 1965. They included Springfield Place, Caledonian Road and Tonbridge Street. The first was part of a bus route connecting Mount Preston with Great George Street and the last was the direct route from the

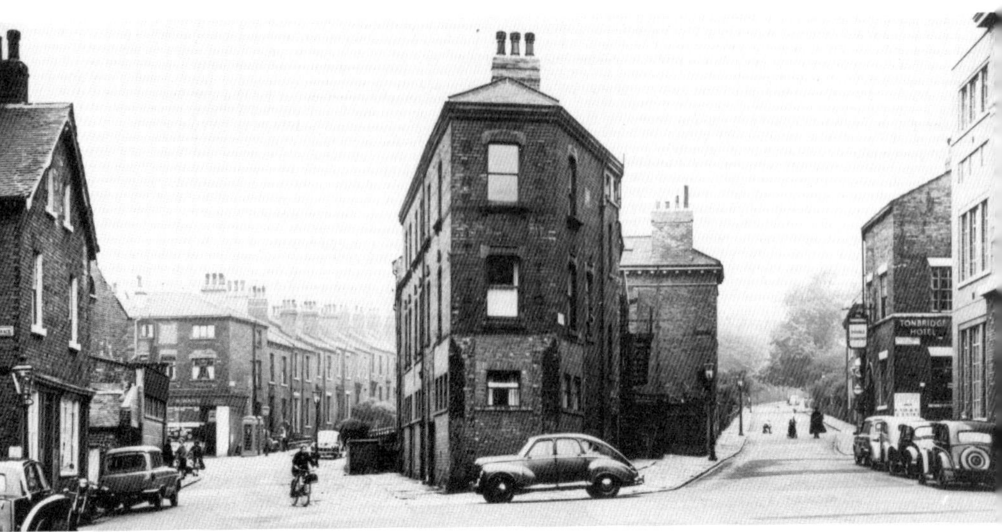

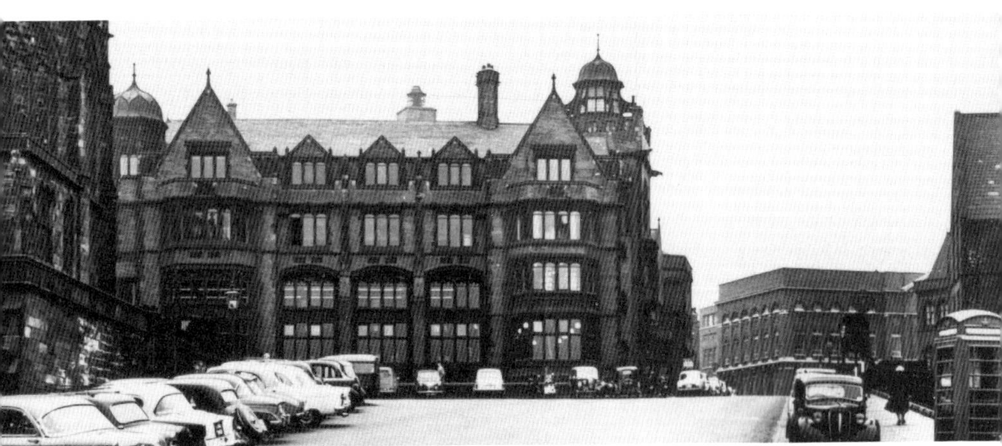

FIG. 33 *Thoresby Place views*
Above: *Caledonian Road, Tonbridge Street, Dental School (right)*
Below: *Looking north — Medical School (left) Dental School and Infirmary (right)*

Medical School to Cavendish Road and to Beech Grove Terrace. Few were sorry to see them go — to this day I can remember the peculiar odour of old dustbins associated with Tonbridge Street, though there was sorrow at the demise of the Tonbridge, a pub at the lower end of the street, which had served many generations of medical students. Fenton Street was closed in the summer of 1964 to allow work on the underpass to begin.[15]

Even before the first plans were published, a complication arose in relation to student numbers. The first sign of this was a request from the UGC in 1962 that the University raise its intake of non-overseas medical students by 10 per cent over the 1960/61 figures and this was accompanied by an ear-marked grant and was agreed without much difficulty.[16] It is interesting to note that the demand for places was considerable; UCCA in October 1963 had 36,100 applications for medicine and there were only 2110 places. However, it must be remembered that each applicant could make up to six applications.[17] Then in January 1964, following the Ministry of Health review of the future need of doctors, in which an overall increase of at least 15 per cent was deemed necessary, the UGC asked the University to consider what growth in intake it was prepared to contemplate over the next five to ten years and requested a reply within five weeks.[18] The Planning Team's Bulletin No 3 had just been issued indicating a bed complement for the new teaching hospital of 1285 on site (955 for acute cases together with 80 psychiatric, 100 geriatric and 150 maternity) and 114 convalescent beds at the Ida Hospital. These figures were based on an annual intake of 108 medical students to give a clinical entry of 100.[19] It was pointed out that this was already a 35 per cent increase over the then intake of 80.

However, before the year was out the UGC had more specifically enquired about a clinical intake of 150 (which would mean a preclinical intake of 162). A national increase of medical graduates from 2220 to 2750 was felt to be necessary, a new school was being set up in Nottingham and it was hoped that an additional 350 places could be provided by six existing medical schools of which Leeds was one.[20]

Additional expansion was viewed in the School with mixed feelings and there was much discussion. It was generally agreed that it was not practicable to increase the number of beds in the Teaching Hospital on the Medical Centre site to provide for more than 100 students, but expansion would be possible by the development of a second independent clinical school or by using the considerable clinical material available at St James's Hospital with radical upgrading of the teaching facilities there to provide a single clinical school based on two hospitals. Others argued that despite any advantages from larger size the great merit of the present plan — all facilities on one site — would be lost; the present plan was already being considered by the Ministry of Health and UGC and renegotiation and replanning would bring considerable delays in the project. The Board of Medicine expressed its support for the original plan and opposition to further expansion, but was overruled by Senate. Senate's Committee had formed the opinion that 'if the Medical School was to expand beyond 100 it might as well expand to provide for an output of 150'.[21] The Regional Hospital Board had already reacted favourably; this was a critical time for St James's and it was important to have a decision within a few months to allow developments already proposed to be modified. Senate believed that the advantages of expansion (eg multiprofessorial units and senior research posts) would be greater than the disadvantages but expansion should be subject to the condition that adequate funds would be available to safeguard quality.[22]

In 1965–66 the University was finding that the announcements of capital building grants for University buildings did not match earlier promises, and many plans had to be revised downwards. Sir Roger Stevens in his statement to Court in November 1966 said 'We still attach very high priority to making a start with the preclinical part of the new Medical School, if funds become available. . . . But by 1969 our building programme will be virtually at a standstill, unless. . . .'[23]

It was obvious that several years must elapse before the Medical Centre could materialise and, because of the urgent need for doctors, plans were made for interim expansion which would allow for an intake of 130 medical students. By March 1967 it was known that £520,000 would be available quickly for this purpose, which involved building an additional section of the Biology Multipurpose building.[24]

In 1970 this building was completed and Physiology moved into it as temporary accommodation, leaving additional space for Anatomy, Pharmacology and the Library in the Thoresby Place School. Some modifications of this space were needed but were quickly and successfully accomplished. Anatomy took over the rooms on the north side; the

Physiology laboratory nearest to the Anatomy theatre formed an excellent, light and airy dissecting room for dental and physiotherapy students — thus leaving the original dissecting room for medicals only. The rooms looking on the Algernon Firth Institute became Pharmacology and Library territory while the rooms of the Professor of Physiology were taken over by the Animal House. Administration and Anatomy had also recently gained space when the men's and women's common rooms moved to the Lipman Building. This was a prefabricated building to the north of the Thoresby Place School, called after Steve Lipman who had been President of the Medical Students' Representative Council, had negotiated for the building and died tragically before it came into use. It was shared by medical and dental students until 1981.

The school was therefore able to accept the first cohort of 130 medical students in October 1970, though one should add that this would not have been possible but for improvements in St James's Hospital with some teaching at Chapel Allerton and Seacroft Hospitals to cope with the additional numbers in the clinical phase. It was a tight squeeze in Anatomy with twenty extra chairs in the lecture theatre, mainly forming an additional back row. Of course there are always a few students who decide rightly or wrongly that lectures are not for them and some of the extra chairs at the front of the theatre soon disappeared.

The demands on the administration were increasing, partly because of the changing size of the school, but also because of the proliferation of committees both within the University and in relation to the Health Service. On Dr Divine's death the post of Sub-Dean lapsed, Dr Sproull was appointed as Senior Administrative Officer and two posts of Clinical Sub-Dean were created, one for the Infirmary and one for St James's. When Mr Pain retired in 1969 it was decided that the Deanship must become a full-time responsibility and Professor D. R. Wood, who had been so heavily involved in the planning of the Medical Centre, was appointed. Mr Lockyer also provided the ongoing influence of a meticulous Secretary to the School.

By the end of 1968 new plans for the Medical Centre had been drawn up but now on the basis of an annual intake of 216 pre-clinical students to give an annual entry of 200 students to the clinical course, in which teaching would be equally divided between the two main hospitals. It was estimated that the total cost of the project would be

£34 million of which £24–25 million would be spent on buildings. Construction would proceed in four phases: Phase I would begin in 1971 and be completed in 1976 to accommodate preclinical departments, departments of Obstetrics and Gynaecology, Paediatrics and Child Health and the Dental School and Hospital. Phases II, III and IV would be completed in 1978, 1981 and 1984 respectively, by which time the Infirmary would be virtually rebuilt.[25] Demolition of the north part of the Thoresby Place School would be necessary for the construction of Phase III but it was intended to preserve the south portion including the main entrance and library, as also the main entrance to the Infirmary to provide with St George's Church a south façade.

Mr Edward Heath laid a marker stone in December 1972 in the garden of the Women's Hospital from which building levels would be taken. Though the site of the Medical and Dental Building did not overlap the Women's Hospital, the latter's operating theatres were so close that either the Women's Hospital must be demolished or the south-east corner of the new building remain uncompleted for a while.

In summer 1973 bridging of the Inner Ring Road commenced and in November the Hospital for Women Outpatients' Department moved to temporary accommodation at 25 Hyde Terrace to be followed in March 1974 by the removal of the remainder of the Hospital to Roundhay Hall. Demolition of the Women's Hospital followed quickly. There were some regrets at its passing for it had been one of the happiest hospitals in Leeds.

The new hospital buildings were being planned with full height service floors between user floors to allow maintenance of services without disturbance of wards. The UGC felt that the cost of this provision could not be justified for the preclinical departments and the Dental School, which would have to conform to the normal practice in University building, with floors at 12 ft intervals and services contained in 3 ft voids above false ceilings. Thus it became necessary to put preclinical departments of the Medical School together with the Dental School and Hospital in a separate building.

REFERENCES

1. Henry Willink, Ministry of Health, Report of the Committee to consider future numbers of medical practitioners and the appropriate intake of medical students 1957.

2. University of Leeds, Development Plan 1960.
3. Teaching Hospital and Medical School, Leeds, Planning Report 1965.
4. University of Leeds *Reporter*, 20 June 1962.
5. New Medical Centre Leeds, Planning Bulletin No 1, November 1962.
6. New Teaching Hospital — Proposed Bed Complement, 17 January 1963.
7. New Medical Centre Leeds, Planning Bulletin No 2, May 1963.
8. University of Leeds *Reporter*, 20 June 1962, p 15.
9. Board of Medicine, Minutes, 21 May 1963.
10. Faculty of Medicine, Planning Committee Minutes, 2 July 1963.
11. Board of Medicine, Minutes, 7 October 1963.
12. Ibid, 19 June 1963.
13. Ibid, 10 December 1963.
14. Ibid, 20 June 1962, p 25.
15. Ibid, 21 October 1964, p 50.
16. University of Leeds *Reporter*, 17 October 1963.
17. Ibid, 25 June 1964.
18. Ibid, 19 February 1964, p 5.
19. Ibid, p 25.
20. Ibid, 16 December 1964.
21. J. V. Loach, 'Notes on Increase in Size of the Medical School', 26 February 1965.
22. University of Leeds *Reporter*, 17 March 1965.
23. Ibid, 16 November 1966.
24. Ibid, 15 March 1967.
25. Ibid, 18 December 1968.

CHAPTER THIRTEEN

The Worsley Medical and Dental Building

AT LAST tangible progress seemed possible. A liaison officer for each department had been appointed in 1970, operational policies had been revised, the arrangement of the space allowed according to UGC schedules (eg 200 sq ft for a lecturer, 600 sq ft for a professor), had been worked out and the furniture, equipment and services for each room settled. The main contract went to John Laing and Son and building commenced in 1974.

A start was made about the same time on the generating station, which was to supply the total energy needs of the whole Medical Centre. It would provide light, heat, electric power, high and low pressure steam, ventilation and cooling, and would house the hospital laundry. It was to use mainly one source of energy and natural gas was chosen: this could be obtained more cheaply on an interruptable supply contract, therefore as a standby energy source two large oil tanks were built into the hillside and the heights of the chimneys raised to reduce the pollution effect of oil-firing. Unfortunately Phase I of the Infirmary which should have started simultaneously was caught by a governmental capital building restriction and its start delayed until June 1977. The cost of the generating station was in the neighbourhood of £4 million, and the authorised expenditure (December 1974) on the Medical and Dental Building was just over £8 million.

The Medical and Dental Building is large, deep, complex, and is built on a sloping site, so that the entrance to the Dental Hospital which is at the west end is one floor above the 'academic entrance' on the north side, which in turn is one floor above the goods and mortuary entrances on the south east. Visitors are sometimes surprised to find on coming through the 'academic entrance' at what they imagine to be ground level, that they are already on Level 4 of the building. This is due to the colour

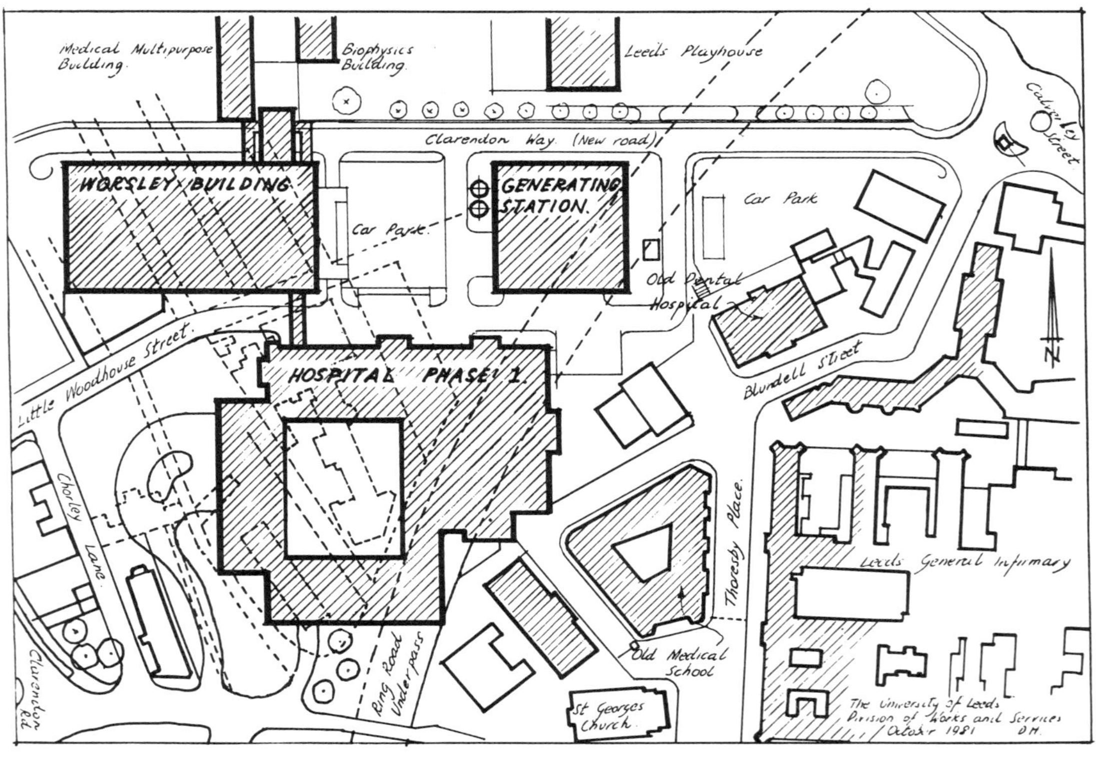

FIG. 34 Site of Worsley Building, Hospital Phase I and Generating Station (former streets, Women's Hospital and Ring Road Underpass shown dotted), drawn by Denys Horner

coding scheme introduced in the Chamberlin Plan in which all levels on the University site are colour coded at 12 ft intervals. The Thoresby Place School on the lowest part of the campus is at Level 1, while the entrance to the Great Hall in University Road is at Level 10 and the Houldsworth School at Level 12.

The arrangement within the building is shown in the following table:

Level 3	beige	Goods entrance. Mortuary entrance. Maintenance workshop.
Level 4	grey	Academic entrance. Porter, locker and cloak rooms.
Level 5	black	Dental Hospital.
Level 6	yellow	School of Dentistry. Audio-visual Services.
Level 7	green	Library. Dean's Office. Administration and Committee rooms. Student and staff common rooms. Medical Lecture Theatre. Medical Illustration.
Level 8	blue	Multidiscipline Laboratories.
Level 9	purple	Anatomy. Pharmacology.
Level 10	red	Physiology. Cardiovascular Studies. Cancer Research.
Level 11	orange	Biochemistry. Radiation Protection and Safety Services.

At level 7 the building communicates by part-open corridor with the Chancellor's Court and this is the main route to other parts of the University. It is also joined to Phase I of the Infirmary by two corridors, one at Dental Hospital level and the other (because of the difference in storey levels in the two buildings) at a landing between Levels 6 and 7 on the S-E staircase. This latter gives good access to the Library and common rooms on the school side and to Clinical Lecture Theatre and dining areas in the hospital.

The building is approximately 330 ft long and 180 ft broad so that in walking round the exterior one covers the best part of a quarter of a mile; because the pattern on each floor even as to the position of corridors is a different one, it is easy to get lost and one then checks as to which floor one is on by looking for the colour code which is usually in sight.

The external finish was intended to be in pale blue brick but these were not available in the quantity needed at the time and so reinforced concrete slabs were used instead.

The rectangular building contains two wells which allow some natural light to internal rooms, but these are partial only, the one in the west half of the building going down as far as Level 9 and the one in the east half to Level 7. The windows in the external walls are an important design feature, for they are narrow and run the entire height of the building, being placed one on each side of a structural pillar, the latter occurring at 15 ft intervals (Fig 35).

Because of the depth of the building the internal rooms had to be air conditioned. There was some discussion about providing external rooms with conventional hot water radiators and opening windows but a decision was taken at an early stage of planning to provide air conditioning throughout with all windows sealed in order to avoid disturbance of air pressures which would interfere with the balance needed for smooth flow of air to all rooms. The only windows which do in fact open are on the staircases. Another feature which sometimes surprises the unitiated is that fume cupboards are not switched on as required but run continuously for they provide the extract of air from the room in which they are sited. Air passes into the rooms through ceiling grilles having passed over heating batteries controlled by room thermostats so that some individual control of room temperature is possible. The narrow windows, though increased in width by 4 in at liaison officers' request were never intended to provide full lighting and except for rooms on the south side on sunny days artificial lighting is almost always necessary. It might seem an over-reaction in design to the enormous areas of glass in the University's Physics/Administration building but it must be remembered that the Medical School was designed in days when energy was expected to be plentiful and cheap. It was to be a prestige building with brilliantly lit corridors and staircases but now many of the fluorescent tubes have been removed. For safety reasons the remaining corridor lighting is not switched off when there is any occupation of the building; there are no individual switches.

Besides the three passenger lifts there are six staircases each communicating with all floors. Access to floors from the staircases (but not vice versa) can be prevented for security reasons, eg at nights. The distances are great and the time taken in the morning for one man to walk round every floor unlocking the staircase doors is said by the head porter, who has tried it, to be an hour. It is possible to go from point A to point B by numerous routes and a game of hide and seek could take a long time.

The Medical Lecture Theatre on Level 7 is well equipped, with facilities for slide projection, overhead projector, 16 mm cine sound, television monitors both for live television (with a camera in the theatre) and for recorded replay and it has large roller blackboards. Lighting can be varied and the acoustics are good; most speakers do not need the

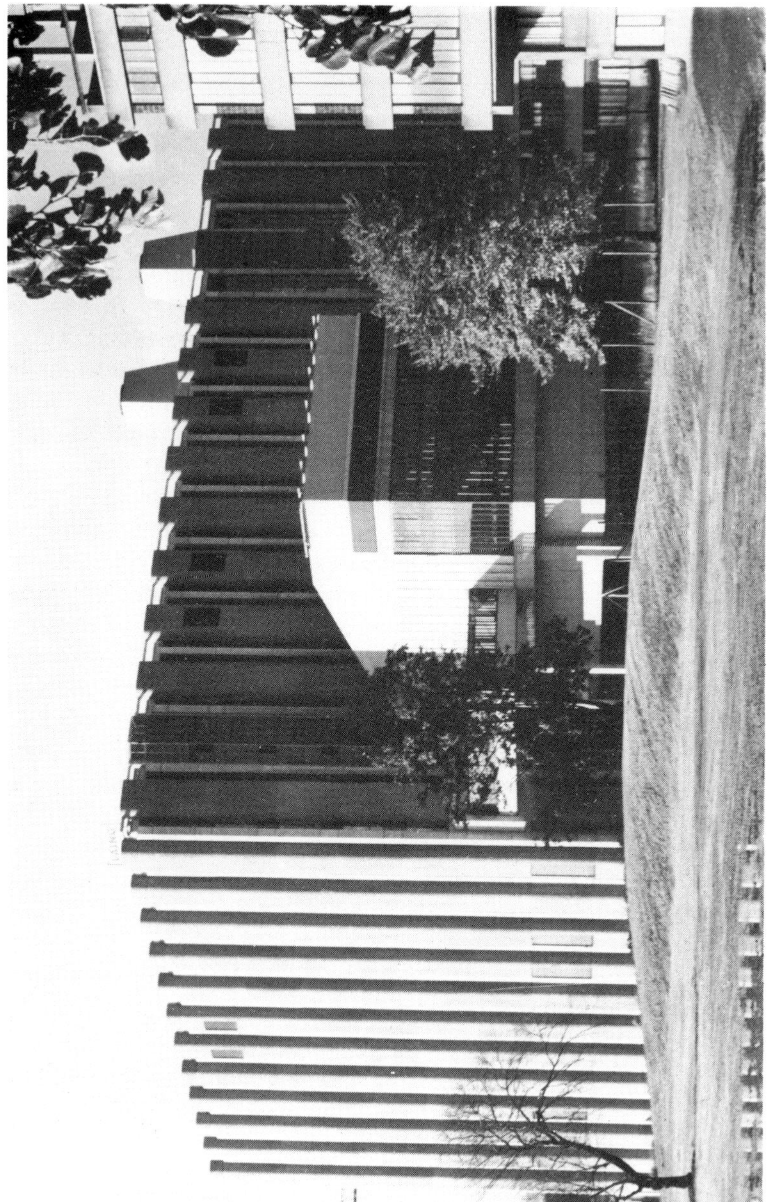

FIG. 35 *Worsley Medical and Dental Building*

public address amplification which is provided. The theatre seats 220; the steep rake of the seating, though not as steep as in the Thoresby Place school, has the effect of bringing the back row nearer to the rostrum and making a large theatre more intimate. The only other lecture theatre in the building is the Dental Lecture Theatre on Level 6, which seats 120 and is similarly equipped. Coffee bars are situated in the common rooms nearby.

As parts of the building were completed, they had to be equipped and furnished. Here tribute must be paid to the Planning Office of the University; in particular to Mr Denys Horner, who was never too busy to answer questions and who by his overall knowledge, his concern for detail and his genial helpfulness enabled this mammoth task to be accomplished smoothly.

The east half of the building was ready first and departments began to move in during the summer of 1977. The move was complex and organised like a military operation. Anatomy moved first, when only two-thirds of its accommodation had been completed; the middle-sized dissecting room was used as a store, members of staff had to share rooms for the first year, complete unpacking was impossible and facilities for research non-existent. However, half the MDLS, sufficient for the first-year students, were ready and this enabled an intake of 160 medical students to be received in October 1977. Other departments moved in at intervals in the succeeding twelve months but the animals not until 1980 when the Home Office Inspector was satisfied about noise levels. There were no such safeguards for humans. The building was officially opened by HRH The Duke of Kent on 23 March 1979 and named the Worsley Medical and Dental Building. A tablet commemorating the opening was unveiled outside the Lecture Theatre on Level 7 (Fig 36). Afterwards the Duke was taken on a brief tour of the building before lunch in University House. In the afternoon honorary degrees were conferred on Sir Robert Bradlaw, former President of the General Dental Council, and on Professor Sir John Walton, Chairman of the Education Committee of the General Medical Council.

In the meantime massive rebuilding had proceeded apace at St James's Hospital, its name changed by Act of Parliament effective on 1 October 1970 to 'St James's University Hospital'. The new buildings are commodious, luxurious in parts, and the hospital is quite transformed. Several University departments have been instituted there and Chairs

The Worsley Medical and Dental Building
Opened by
His Royal Highness the Duke of Kent
23 March 1979

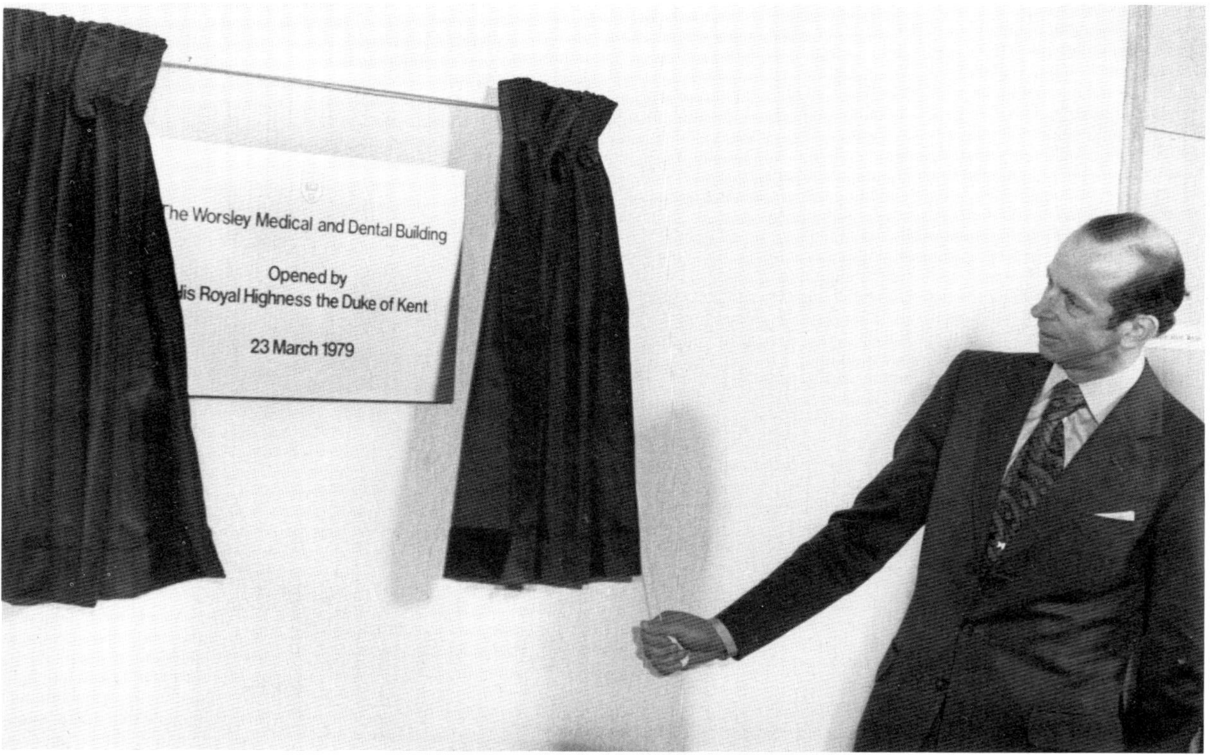

FIG. 36 *The Opening of the New School by HRH the Duke of Kent*

established in Medicine (1970), Surgery (1973), Obstetrics and Gynaecology (1973), Psychiatry (1979), Paediatrics and Child Health (1980), and Orthopaedic Surgery (1981).

The Clinical Sciences Building which houses all the University departments at St James's (except Obstetrics which is incorporated in the hospital) together with teaching and tutorial rooms and a small library, was started in 1976. The topping out ceremony was performed by Professor D. R. Wood on 17 July 1978. The cost of the building had been £2.4 million. It is centrally situated on the St James's site and should make a most important contribution to training in the clinical phase.

Phase I of the Infirmary, which had a late start in 1977, is being built by the Shepherd Haden Young consortium and is now on schedule. The topping out ceremony was performed by Sir William Tweddle in December 1980. It should be ready for commissioning in the late summer of 1982.

The Medical School in Thoresby Place is also undergoing a radical but most successful transformation and updating, to house the Department of Microbiology and a part of the Department of Chemical Pathology. The Entrance Hall, Library and Board Room have been retained structurally unaltered, the Library providing a home for the University Archives, and the Board Room for a departmental library; new laboratories at corridor level have replaced the general lecture theatre; the dissecting room has become a laboratory but is undivided; a lift has been installed; old awkward staircases have gone, new corridors have appeared, and tutorial rooms have been built on a new floor above the annexe, while the old refectory, it seems by poetic justice, now houses a 'media kitchen' for Microbiology. The Algernon Firth Institute will shortly be vacated to be upgraded to meet the modern needs of the Department of Pathology.

The whole medical centre project has been one of great complexity involving a great deal of consultation and compromise and generating several filing cabinets completely full of paper, the latter providing a daunting task for any future historian. It is hardly surprising that there have been grumbles, but advantage lies in that there is now adequate space for work and there are still empty shelves in the library.

CHAPTER FOURTEEN

Retrospect and Prospect

THE LEEDS SCHOOL OF MEDICINE has had five homes, each bigger than the previous one. The last three have been purpose-built, imaginative in conception, advanced in design for their time and all were late in being finished. After a time students have developed an affection for the buildings and this has been particularly true of Thoresby Place.

However, it is not in buildings alone that the spirit of a school lies, but rather in the individuals who have worked in it. From faltering beginnings, when it was not certain that the School could survive, when other schools after a transient existence were closing, the early pioneers of the Leeds School went forward in independence and faith, wary of pitfalls, giving time and energy that could often ill be spared from their relatively short lives, in order to ensure that the School was successful.

The School has been fortunate from its earliest days in the calibre of the men who have served it: the Heys, the Teales, Thackrah, the Smiths, the Nunneleys, the Braithwaites, Heaton, Scattergood, Allbutt, Jessop, McGill, Mayo-Robson, Littlewood, Moynihan, Dobson, Flint, and others more recently who have pioneered advances in their profession; it has been fortunate too in those who have devoted themselves, in a less spectacular way, to the well being of the School from Garlick, Scattergood and Jamieson onwards; fortunate in the development of the Yorkshire College, in which one of its own men, Dr Heaton, played so large a part; and in being steered into union with the College by Heaton, Scattergood and Allbutt, and in having a succession of excellent Deans active in College and University affairs.

The School has grown continuously, if somewhat spasmodically over the century and a half of its existence, but the doubling in size during the decade 1970–80 has meant more adjustment for more people. Tradition takes time to develop and make its imprint on new buildings. But a start has been made. Corners of the Worsley Building have been humanised;

photographs have appeared on the walls of the corridors even if in some cases they are merely those of the staff of the adjacent department.

Attempts are made to ensure that every student joins a small tutorial group, is known at least to some members of staff and is not just a computer number. Clinical teaching still occurs in 'firms' and continues on a personal level. The traditional friendliness of Leeds welcomes new students at an annual reception; refreshments, wine and strawberries are consumed after the degree ceremony at the end of the course. It shows through too in the good relations which the oldest part of the University — a part which has for long remained geographically separate and is now much more closely integrated — enjoys with other departments and the central administration, sited further north on the campus.

Prior to the celebrations of the 150th anniversary a copy of the School shield and motto has been placed in the Entrance Hall at Level 4 of the Worsley Building. The original is to be found in the Hexagon Entrance Hall of the Thoresby Place School, there in Burmantofts tiling (Fig 22). The shield is red with a gold chevron on which is seen a serpent in natural colour. In the upper part of the shield are 'the blazing suns of York' adopted by Edward IV on his badge and below is the golden fleece of Leeds. The shield is surmounted by a gold sphinx on a wreath, gold and red. The motto was chosen by Mr Scattergood who was Dean in Yorkshire College days when the Thoresby Place School was built (see p 85). The copy has been expertly finished and those who examine it carefully may see that the specialist painter who completed the work has signed his name on the open book carried by an angel at the end of the inscription.

William Hey, a founder of Leeds General Infirmary, is said to have drawn no distinction between rich and poor. Moynihan preached gentleness in examination of patients, and the 'caressing of tissues'. These are ideals on which the best medical practice is based and in spite of changes the traditions of the past are still alive in Leeds.

One wonders whether the remaining Phases of the Medical Centre will ever be built as originally conceived in the development plan, whether the planned expansion to an intake of 216 medical students will ever materialise. The unfolding of the next fifty years will give the answer.

APPENDIX I

List of Members of Council and Lecturers at the Leeds School of Medicine 1831-84*

ELECTED		RETIRED
Founders 1831	Dr Williamson	October 1839
	Dr Hunter	June 1842
	Mr Smith	July 1867
	Mr Wm Hey	July 1857
	Mr T. P. Teale	July 1851
	Mr Garlick	July 1853
	Dr Disney L. Thorp	March 1837
	Mr Thackrah	Died May 1833
	Mr Price	June 1853
	Mr John Hey	Died 1837
1835	Mr Thos Nunneley	July 1865
	Mr Geo Morley	August 1862
1837	Mr Wildsmith	Died August 1839
	Mr Nelson	December 1840
1839	Dr Chadwick	August 1871
	Dr G. P. Smith	July 1868
1841	Mr Braithwaite	August 1862
	Mr Saml Hey	August 1870
	Mr J. I. Ikin	July 1866
	Mr S. Wilkinson	June 1843
1842	Mr S. Radcliffe	August 1849
	Dr Drennan	July 1844
1843	Mr S. Staniland	Died February 1850
1844	Dr Heaton	July 1878
1851	Mr W. N. Price	July 1870, re-elected 1875 — August 1884
	Mr T. Scattergood	†
	Mr C. G. Wheelhouse	July 1875
	Dr Thos Clarke	August 1854

1854	Dr Ed Bishop	August 1864
1856	Mr T. Pridgin Teale	May 1876
	Mr Wm Hall	July 1875
1861	Dr Hardwick	Died 1864
1862	Mr Ed Atkinson	†
	Mr Jas Seaton	1874
1864	Dr T. Clifford Allbutt	August 1884
1866	Dr R. T. Land	July 1879
	Mr Jessop	†
	Mr J. A. Nunneley	†
1868	Dr J. E. Eddison	†
1870	Mr Chas J. Wright	†
	Mr James Walker	August 1883
1872	Mr Oglesby	July 1876
1874	Mr John Horsfall	1883
	Mr Edmund Robinson	†
1875	Mr A. F. McGill	†
	Dr James Braithwaite	†
1877	Dr Churton	†
1878	Mr A. W. M. Robson	†
1882	Dr E. H. Jacob	†

* Taken from a published list with handwritten additions in Leeds Medical School Prospectuses 1864–84.

† Became professors and lecturers in the Yorkshire College.

APPENDIX II

List of Presidents, Treasurers and Secretaries of the Leeds School of Medicine 1831–84; and of Medical Deans in the Yorkshire College and the University of Leeds

PRESIDENTS

1831–32	Dr Williamson	1856–57	Mr Morley
1832–33	Dr Williamson	1857–58	Mr Wm Braithwaite
1833–34	Dr Williamson	1858–59	Dr Heaton
1834–35	Mr S. Smith	1859–60	Mr W. Nicholson Price
1835–36	Dr Hunter	1860–61	Mr Scattergood
1836–37	Mr Wm Hey (the third)	1861–62	Mr Wheelhouse
1837–38	Mr Wm Price	1862–63	Dr Chadwick
1838–39	Dr Williamson	1863–64	Mr S. Smith
1839–40	Mr S. Smith	1864–65	Mr T. Nunneley
1840–41	Dr Hunter	1865–66	Mr Samuel Hey
1841–42	Mr T. P. Teale	1866–67	Mr Samuel Hey
1842–43	Mr T. Nunneley	1867–68	Mr T. Pridgin Teale, Jr
1843–44	Dr Chadwick	1868–69	Mr Hall
1844–45	Dr Pyemont Smith	1869–70	Mr Seaton
1845–46	Mr Wm Hey (the third)	1870–71	Mr Atkinson
1846–47	Mr Wm Braithwaite	1871–72	Dr Allbutt
1847–48	Mr Ikin	1872–73	Dr Heaton
1848–49	Mr Samuel Hey	1873–74	Mr Scattergood
1849–50	Mr Morley	1874–75	Mr Wheelhouse
1850–51	Dr Heaton	1875–76	Mr Jessup
1851–52	Dr Chadwick	1876–77	Dr Land
1852–53	Mr T. Nunneley	1877–78	Mr John A. Nunneley
1853–54	Mr S. Smith	1878–79	Dr Eddison
1854–55	Mr Ikin	1879–80	Mr Atkinson
1855–56	Dr Pyemont Smith	1880–81	Mr Wright

1881–82 Mr W. Nicholson Price
1882–83 Mr Walker
1883–84 Dr Allbutt

TREASURERS

1831–53 Mr Garlick
1853–65 Mr Samuel Hey
1865–79 Dr Heaton
1879–84 Mr Scattergood

SECRETARIES

1831–39 Mr T. P. Teale
1839–44 Mr Morley
1844–50 Mr Staniland
1850–56 Dr Pyemont Smith
1856–59 Mr W. Nicholson Price
1859–62 Mr Wheelhouse
1862–64 Dr Hardwick
1864–70 Mr Atkinson
1870–78 Dr Eddison
1878–80 Mr Wright
1880–84 Mr Horsfall

MEDICAL DEANS OF THE YORKSHIRE COLLEGE (UP TO 1904) AND OF THE UNIVERSITY OF LEEDS (FROM 1904)

1884–1900 Mr T. Scattergood
1900–07 Professor de Burgh Birch
1907–13 Professor A. S. Grünbaum
1913–17 Professor de Burgh Birch
1917–18 Professor J. B. Hellier
1918–35 Professor J. K. Jamieson
1935–41 Mr H. Collinson
1941–49 Professor M. J. Stewart
1949–52 Professor J. W. McLeod
1952–60 Professor P. J. Moir
1960–69 Mr A. B. Pain
1969– Professor D. R. Wood

APPENDIX III

Former Professors and Heads of Departments in the Yorkshire College and in the University of Leeds

A. IN THE YORKSHIRE COLLEGE* (1884–1904)

Anatomy	
A. F. McGill	1884–87
T. W. Griffith	1887–1904
Physiology	
De Burgh Birch	1884–1904
Pathology	
E. H. Jacob	1884–94
E. F. Trevelyan	1894–1904
Medicine	
J. E. Eddison	1884–98
A. G. Barrs	1898–1904
Surgery	
T. R. Jessop	1884–87
A. F. McGill	1887–90
A. W. Mayo-Robson	1890–99
E. Ward	1899–1904
Ophthalmology	
J. A. Nunneley	1884–95 non-professorial
Ophthalmology and Otology	
H. Secker Walker	1895–1904 non-professorial
Midwifery	
C. J. Wright	1884–88 non-professorial
C. J. Wright	1888–1904

* Abstracted from the Calendars of the Yorkshire College 1884–1904.

Diseases of Women and Children

Jas Braithwaite	1884–1889 non-professorial
J. B. Hellier	1889–1904 non-professorial

Materia Medica, Pharmacology and Therapeutics

J. B. Hellier	1884–89 non-professorial
A. G. Barrs	1889–94 non-professorial
A. G. Barrs	1894–98
C. M. Chadwick	1898–1904

Forensic Medicine

T. Scattergood	1884–1900 non-professorial
with C. M. Chadwick	1889–98 non-professorial
H. J. Campbell	1898–1904 non-professorial

Mental Diseases

W. Bevan Lewis	1885–1904 non-professorial

Hygiene

R. N. Hartley	1884–1904 non-professorial

B. IN THE UNIVERSITY OF LEEDS* (FROM 1904)

Anatomy

T. W. Griffith	1904–10
J. K. Jamieson	1910–36
A. Durward	1936–64

Physiology

De Burgh Birch	1904–17
H. S. Raper	1917–23
W. F. Shanks	1923–26
B. A. McSwiney	1926–36
A. Hemmingway	1936–67

Biochemistry

F. C. Happold	1946–67
P. N. Campbell	1967–75

* Abstracted from the University of Leeds Calendar 1981–82 and re-arranged.

Pathology and Bacteriology

A. S. Leyton	1904–17
M. J. Stewart (pathology)	1918–50
J. W. McLeod (bacteriology)	1922–52
R. A. Willis (pathology)	1950–55
C. E. Lumsden (pathology)	1956–74

Bacteriology

C. L. Oakley	1952–72

Microbiology

K. S. Zinnemann (clinical bacteriology)	1970–73

Chemical Pathology

F. S. Fowweather	1946–56
G. H. Lathe	1957–77

Clinical Investigation

P. Fourman	1963–68

Experimental Pathology and Cancer Research

R. D. Passey	1926–53
H. N. Green	1954–67
D. B. Clayson	1967–74

Medicine

A. G. Barrs	1904–10
T. W. Griffith	1910–25
W. H. M. Telling	1925–32
G. W. Watson	1932–37
W. MacAdam	1937–46
F. F. Hellier (dermatology)	1968–69
Sir Ronald Tunbridge	1946–71
G. P. McNicol (LGI)	1971–81

Clinical Medicine

A. G. Barrs	1910–20
G. W. Watson	1925–32
R. A. Veale	1933–34
W. MacAdam	1934–37
J. L. F. C. Burrow	1937–48
S. J. Hartfall	1948–64

Surgery

H. Littlewood	1904–10
R. L Knaggs	1910–19
B. G. A. Moynihan	1925–27
J. F. Dobson	1927–33
H. Collinson	1933–36
E. R. Flint	1936–40
D. Chamberlain	1946–56
J. C. Goligher	1954–77

Clinical Surgery

B. G. A. Moynihan	1910–25
J. F. Dobson	1925–27
H. Collinson	1927–33
A. Richardson	1933–34
E. R. Flint	1934–36
L. R. Braithwaite	1936–38
H. W. Symons	1940–56
P. J. Moir	1952–60
D. Chamberlain	1956–61

Urological Surgery

L. N. Pyrah	1956–64

Orthopaedic Surgery

J. M. P. Clark	1968–72

Anaesthesia

R. P. Harbord	1947–63 non-professorial
J. F. Nunn	1964–68

Obstetrics and Gynaecology

C. J. Wright	1904–08
J. B. Hellier	1908–18
E. O. Croft	1918–23
Carlton Oldfield	1923–30
William Gough	1931–36
A. M. Claye	1936–61

Diseases of Children
C. W. Vining 1922–27 non-professorial
C. W. Vining 1927–46

Paediatrics and Child Health
W. S. M. Craig 1946–68

Radiology
A. S. Johnstone 1948–68

Radio Diagnosis
M. S. F. McLachlan 1973–76

Radiotherapy
P. B. Kunkler 1968–72

Medical Physics
F. W. Spiers 1950–72

Mineral Metabolism
B. E. C. Nordin 1970–81

Pharmacology and Therapeutics
E. F. Trevelyan 1904–05 non-professorial
E. F. Trevelyan 1905–08
H. J. Campbell 1908–19
R. A. Veale 1925–32
S. J. Hartfall 1937–48

Pharmacology
W. A. Bain 1946–59
D. R. Wood 1960–69

Mental Diseases
W. Bevan Lewis 1904–08 non-professorial
W. Bevan Lewis 1908–10
J. Shaw Bolton 1911–34
M. J. McGrath 1935–46 non-professorial

Psychiatry
H. V. Dicks 1946–48
D. R. MacCalman 1948–57

G. R. Hargreaves	1955–62
M. Hamilton	1964–77

Forensic Medicine

H. J. Campbell	1904–08
F. W. Eurich	1908–32
W. H. M. Telling	1932–38
P. L. Sutherland	1938–46
C. J. Polson	1947–69

Public Health

J. S. Cameron	1904–15
W. Angus	1917–19
J. J. Jervis	1920–47
I. G. Davies	1947–58
D. B. Bradshaw	1958–73

Dentistry

T. Talmage Read (clinical dental surgery)	1931–59
D. Jackson (children's and preventative dentistry)	1965–80
S. M. Weidmann (oral biology)	1965–69

APPENDIX IV

Two Extracts from the Inaugural Lecture by James Paget, FRS, at the Opening of the Park Street School in 1865

I need hardly say that the possession of knowledge and the power of using it are very different things; men differ scarcely more in the one than in the other; and often, in the hurry of life's business, one sees reason to believe that a little knowledge always in hand is better than much more which is far off or unwieldy. Certainly, it is so in examinations. Two men, suppose of unequal knowledge, go in together. The one who has least, produces what he has at once and to the point; the other does not: he could do it tomorrow, but not today; or he could write a book, but he cannot answer questions; so the one passes, and the other is plucked.

And this result is not altogether unjust (I do not say it is right, but it is not entirely wrong). For the examination for a diploma is but one instance of that constant subjection to tests in which a great part of our whole life is spent, and in which knowledge scarcely deserves the name, if if cannot be produced in the right time and place. In this view, every emergency of practice is like a stern examiner, requiring a right swift answer; and nothing is more striking than the way in which, with practice, men learn to give in their replies. When men grow wiser as they grow older, it is not only that they are always gathering knowledge, but that they are always becoming more able to use their knowledge readily and aptly. A great deal of the fruit of experience is not so much the learning to do better as the learning to do well more easily.

Think of this, always, as one of the collateral advantages of the very frequent examinations which I am recommending. They are not only the best means, and to many the indispensable means, for insuring the ready use of the knowledge requisite for a safe final passage, but they are the best that you can have for practice in the art of thinking during anxiety and other mental troubles. He that has learnt to think and to speak correctly in an emergency is already far on his way to success in life.

Coolness in operating, and in the various difficulties of surgical and obstetric practice, is sure to be an object of your admiration; but its advantages in these parts of our profession only seem greater — they are not really greater — than in the wider duties of advising and prescribing. In every part and time of life, self-possession — that is, the power of thinking is the midst of distracting forces — is one of the best possessions that a man can have.

* * * *

We are all too apt to forget the difference between seeing and observing, between hearing and learning; too apt to give ourselves to mere sight-seeing, and to think that we are studying when we are only gratifying our curiosity in seeing or hearing strange things. Now, our natural curiosity need not be suppressed; for, expecially among students, it augments activity; but it should not be a chief motive with us — it should not guide us — for it always lacks discretion and that steady singleness of purpose by which all work should be directed. Remember, then, when you are seeing practice, that you will learn little from it, unless with a clear act of the attention you look and observe, and then study and reflect on what you have observed, and so turn it into knowledge; and then store the knowledge in its right place. Without this you may be always in the wards, and yet gain no more real knowledge of practice than they who are always reading or hearing lectures.

And while thus urging you to the habit of careful observation, let me recommend to you, as one of the best means of cultivating it, the custom of recording your observations. . . . What would you expect of a young artist who would only draw in the evening from the memory of people seen for a few minutes in the course of the day? Why, you might expect just what you may find in many cases and descriptions written on the same plan: mere caricatures and deceptive outlines of the truth. Write from nature (and draw from nature, too, if you can); and do it not only that you have records for later study, but that you may learn to observe exactly and profoundly. For, as a good artist sees much more — really sees more — in a face or in a landscape than other people do, so does he who has the habit of looking earnestly at objects that he may describe them, or paint them in words.

Index